MANUAL OF HISTOLOGICAL TECHNIQUES AND HISTOLOGICAL AND ULTRASTRUCTURAL FEATURES OF SOME ENDOCRINE GLANDS

C.K.MANNA

Published by New Generation Publishing in 2024

Copyright © C.K.MANNA 2024

First Edition

The author asserts the moral right under the Copyright, Designs and Patents Act 1988 to be identified as the author of this work.

All Rights reserved. No part of this publication may be reproduced, stored in a retrieval system or transmitted, in any form or by any means without the prior consent of the author, nor be otherwise circulated in any form of binding or cover other than that which it is published and without a similar condition being imposed on the subsequent purchaser.

ISBN: 978-1-83563-095-2

www.newgeneration-publishing.com
New Generation Publishing

Dedication

For my Dad, ------

No one has ever been given more loving and unconditional support than I have been given by you.

I love you, too.

Dr. C.K.Manna

Acknowledgement

No one who achieves success does so without acknowledging the help of others. The wise and confident acknowledge this help with gratitude.

Alfred North Whitehead

The man of science is a poor philosopher.

Albert Einstein

Writing a book is harder than I thought and more rewarding than I could have ever imagined. None of this would have been possible without the help of some persons. He stood by me during every struggle and all my successes. That is true friendship.

Considering the ideas of the **Eminent Personalities** I would like to acknowledge some persons who directly or indirectly helped me a lot to write this type of book on the "MANUAL OF HISTOLOGICAL TECHNIQUES AND HISTOLOGICAL AND ULTRASTRUCTURAL FEATURES OF SOME ENDOCRINE GLANDS."

I would also like to give special thanks to my wife (Dr. Samita Manna) and my family as a whole for their continuous support and understanding when undertaking my research and writing my book.

Finally, I would like to thank God, for letting me through all the difficulties. I have experienced your guidance dy by day. You are the one who let me finish my degree. I will keep on trusting you for my future.

Dr. C.K.Manna

Professor (Retired)

University of Kalyani, Nadia, W.B., INDIA

PREFACE

The development of this subject (i.e., **Histology and Histopathology**) is based on the premise that histology is more than knowing the anatomy and physiology of tissues - it also involves developing the practical ability to systematically examine tissues microscopically.

Histology, branch of biology concerned with the composition and structure of plant and animal tissues in relation to their specialized functions. The terms histology and microscopic anatomy are sometimes used interchangeably, but a fine distinction can be drawn between the two studies. The fundamental aim of histology is to determine how tissues are organized at all structural levels, from cells and intercellular substances to organs.

In their investigations, histologists mainly examine quantities of tissue that have been removed from the living body ; these tissues are cut into very thin, almost transparent slices using a special cutting instrument known as a microtome. These thin sections, as they are called, may then be stained with various dyes to increase the contrast between their various cellular components so that the latter can be more easily resolved using an optical microscope.

The origin of the term "special stains" is unknown, but one can be certain that it began to be used after **1876** when the combination of **haematoxylin and eosin** (H & E) was introduced and soon became the oversight method of first choice for most practitioners of normal histology and histopathology. The "special stain" terminology is most commonly used in the clinical environment, and simply means any technique other than the **H & E** method that is used to impart colours to a specimen.

On the other hand, the H & E stain is the most popular staining method in histology and medical diagnosis laboratories. Although **H & E** is very popular among histotechnologists and pathologists for looking at biopsies and surgical and post mortem specimens, the method has some limitations. For example, **H & E** does not identify microorganisms (e.g., H. pylori), or for that matter, specific tissue molecules in cancers (e.g., glycoproteins or **glycosaminoglycans**) or abnormal increase of interstitial fibres in some neoplastic clonal proliferations of the haematopoietic stem cell diseases (e.g., myelodysplastic syndromes).

Both **H & E** and special stains may be applied either manually or through automated methods using specialized instruments.

Many of the methods were developed in some other Special Stains Laboratory and have been published in various journals including **The Journal of Histotechnology, Stain Technology, Biotechnic and Histochemistry, Laboratory Medicine and Theory and Practice of Histological Techniques.**

. It is mostly a descriptive discipline that uses light and electron microscopy to describe tissue morphology. The anatomy and organization of tissues are essential to understand the normal physiology and pathology of the organs. Histopathology is a branch of histology that deals with alterations and diseases of tissues.

Ultra structure (or **ultra-structure**) is the architecture of cells and biomaterials that is visible at higher magnifications than found on a standard optical light microscope. This traditionally meant the resolution and magnification range of a conventional transmission electron microscope (**TEM**) when viewing biological specimens such as cells, tissue, or organs. Ultra structure can also be viewed with scanning electron microscopy and super-resolution microscopy, although **TEM** is a standard histology technique for viewing ultra structure.

In 1931, German engineers Max Knoll and Ernst Ruska invented the first electron microscope. With the development and invention of this microscope, the range of observable structures that were able to be explored and analyzed increased immensely, as biologists became progressively interested in the sub microscopic organization of cells. This new area of research concerned itself with substructure, also known as the **ultra structure**.

TEM is a microscopy technique whereby an electron beam is transmitted through an ultra-thin specimen. As the electron beam passes through, it interacts with the specimen. The image gets formed from the interaction of electrons transmitted through a plastic-embedded specimen. The obtained image is magnified and focused onto an imaging device like Fluorescent screen, on a layer of photographic film, or to be detected by a sensor such as a CCD camera. TEM enables the resolution and visualization of detail that is not apparent through light microscopy, even when light microscopy is combined with immune-histochemical analysis.

Despite remarkable new techniques, the greatest source of error in thin sections for TEM still lies in sample preparation. In conventional fixation and embedment in epoxy resins at ambient temperature, organelle structure and spatial arrangements of macromolecular complexes rapidly change after tissue sampling. For example, the cytoskeleton, Golgi complex, and endomembrane system are remodelled within fractions of a second after tissue anoxia. This requires attention to sample collection, especially times of sampling, trimming, and temperature of fixatives and buffers for fixation.

After discussion with various **Students , Scientists and Endocrinologists** in this relevant field, it seems that there are no specific books - for the study of **histology** and **ultra structural** details of the major endocrine glands. Considering the lacuna , a systematic approach has been made by me for the benefit of the **students, research workers and Scientists** of various Disciplines. Hope this book will be quite helpful to the **Students and Research workers and Teachers** in this specific field.

CHAPTER – I

BASIC HISTOLOGICAL AND ULTRASTRUCTURAL TECHNIQUES

Introduction

Histology is the branch of anatomy that focuses on the study of the finer structures of animals and plants with a microscope, started to emerge as a distinct discipline within the biological and medical sciences during the early part of the nineteenth century.

Although one may divide microscopic anatomy into *organology*, the study of organs, *histology*, the study of tissues, and cytology, the study of cells, modern usage places all of these topics under the field of histology. In medicine, histopathology is the branch of histology that includes the microscopic identification and study of diseased tissue. In the field of paleontology, the term paleohistology refers to the histology of fossil organisms.

The word "histology" stems from the Greek word "histos," meaning web or tissue, and "logia," meaning branch of learning. In brief, histological processing involves obtaining fresh tissue, preserving it (i.e., fixing it) in order to allow it to remain in as life-like a state as possible, cutting it into very thin sections (3–8 microns), mounting it on glass microscopic slides, and then staining the sections so that they can be observed under a microscope to identify different histological components within the tissue. The term tissue refers typically to a collection of cells.

Hematoxylin and eosin (H&E stain) is one of the most commonly used stains in histology to show the general structure of the tissue. Hematoxylin stains cell nuclei blue; eosin, an acidic dye, stains the cytoplasm and other tissues in different stains of pink.

Father of Histology

Histology, the study of details of tissues, came into usage in the 1700s by the scientist Marie François Xavier Bichat. Bichat is now considered to be the father of modern histology and descriptive anatomy. Bichat's work on 21 tissues was all based on gross dissection rather than the usage of the microscope . Prior to that, Marcello Malpighi was the first scientist to observe capillaries, and thus was considered to be the true "Father of Histology" . It was only until 1819 that Mayer coined the term "Histology". He combined two Greek root words that are histos, for tissues, and logos, for study. Histos originally was to describe any woven material, until Sir Richard Owen suggested the large usage of it in 1844 .

Histology today

Performing histology today is a much different experience than it was at the turn of the 20th century. It was then that paraffin wax and formalin were first employed to embed and fix tissues, respectively, with the invention of a microtome capable of sectioning animal tissue occurring slightly earlier, in 1848. Important additions have also been made to histology procedures within the last several decades, such as the use of antibodies to stain tissue sections in a process called immunohistochemistry that was first described in the 1980s. Scientists have also turned to automation to process a larger number of samples with greater speed and precision and to perform multiple kinds of stains simultaneously. This rise in sample number has also led to the need for chemical resistant histology grade labels, to ensure samples are properly and securely identified. As the biomedical research industry evolves, so too does histological analysis, as it continually responds to new scientific and medical challenges for a growing (and aging) worldwide population.

Some recent conversations I have had got me thinking about bioscience students and their first encounter with the word and the world of 'histology'. In pursuing the study of biology and carving out a career in the life sciences, many of us will no doubt need (or want) to use histology in our studies and research.

So, what exactly is histology ? And how has it developed over the years? Find out as we take a paddle into the history of histology.

The word 'histology' basically means 'tissue science'. The history and evolution of histology go hand-in-hand with that of microscopy - obviously, there is not much need for histology without microscopy!

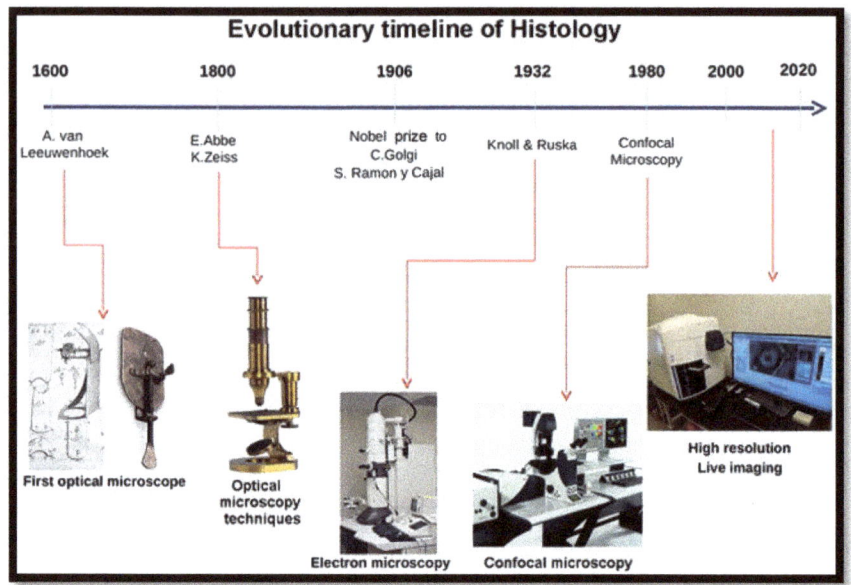

Fig. 1. Timeline of the milestones that marked the evolution of Histology.

In the 19th century histology was an academic discipline in its own right. The French anatomist Xavier Bichat introduced the concept of tissue in anatomy in 1801, and the term "histology" (German: Histologie), coined to denote the "study of tissues", first appeared in a book by Karl Meyer in 1819.

Definition of Fixation

It is a complex series of chemical events which brings about changes in the various chemical constituents of cell like hardening, however the cell morphology and structural detail is preserved. Unless a tissue is fixed soon after the removal from the body it will undergo degenerative changes due to autolysis and putrefaction so that the morphology of the individual cell will be lost.

Aims and Effects of fixation

If a fresh tissue is kept as such at room temperature, it will become liquefied with a foul odour mainly due to action of bacteria i.e. , putrefaction and autolysis so the first and fore most aim of fixation is :
1. To preserve the tissue in as If like manner as possible.
2. To prevent post-mortem changes like autolysis and putrefaction.

Autolysis is the lysis or dissolution of cells by enzymatic action probably as a result of rupture of lysosomes.

Putrefaction : The breakdown of tissue by bacterial action often with formation of gas.

3. Preservation of chemical compounds and micro anatomic constituents so that further histochemistry is possible.
4. *Hardening* : the hardening effect of fixatives allows easy manipulation of soft tissue like brain, intestines etc.
5. *Solidification*: Converts the normal semi fluid consistency of cells (gel) to an irreversible semisolid consistency (solid).
6. *Optical differentiation* - it alters to varying degrees the refractive indices of the various components of cells and tissues so that unstained components are more easily visualized than when unfixed.
7. *Effects of staining* - certain fixatives like formaldehyde intensifies the staining character of tissue especially with haematoxylin.

What is fixation

Fixation is a process in which cells or tissue are fixed in physical state and partly in chemical state so that they will withstand subsequent treatment with various reagents with a minimum loss, distortion or decomposition.

What is the principle in the action of fixative

Fixatives act by denaturing or precipitating proteins which then form a meshwork due to cross linking of proteins. This meshwork tends to hold the other cell constituents in vivo relation to each other and insoluble proteins provide mechanical strength for subsequent procedures.

What is an ideal fixative

Ideal fixative should :
  a) Penetrate tissue quickly
  b) Rapid in action
  c) Isotonic
  d) Cause minimum loss and minimum physical and chemical alteration of the tissue and its components
  e) Cheap, stable and safe to use.

TYPE OF FIXATION

Immersion/in vitro
Perfusion/in vivo
Vapour
Spray/coating
Freeze drying
Microwave fixation

Immersion and Perfusion Fixation

Immersion. In the immersion method, samples of tissues are plunged into fixative solutions. It is also used for blood smears or for fixing sections obtained from unfixed frozen samples. Some precautions should be kept in mind:

1) The piece of tissue should not be larger than 0.5 cm in thickness to allow the fixative enters the deeper part of the sample before the cells start to get damaged. Penetration speed depends on the fixative type and the tissue to be fixed. The size of the sample should be considered according to the fixative type. Slow diffusion fixatives are recommended in samples not larger than 0.2 cm. Tissue features need to be considered. For example, fixation penetration is faster in loose tissues or samples with large spaces for diffusion.

2) The volume of the fixative needs to be 10 to 20 times larger than the volume of the sample.

3) Osmolarity of the sample and the fixative solution need as similar as possible.

4) The pH of the fixative solution should be close to the physiological pH of the sample.

5) For a similar type of sample, fixation time depends on fixative features: diffusion and fixation (intensity and speed of making bridges between proteins or how quick proteins coagulate). The fixation time must be enough for a proper fixation, but not excessive because it may cause artifacts in the sample. A gentle agitation of the sample during fixation is recommended for increasing the fixative penetration, which reduces the fixation time. 24 hours of fixation is common for most of the fixatives. However, for some of them, like formaldehyde, fixation time may last for a week.

Perfusion. In this fixation method, the fixative solution is introduced through the vascular system and reach all the cells of the tissue via capillary net. It is possible to fix a whole animal if the fixative solution enters through the left ventricle of the heart. Then, the fixative solution is driven through the vascular branches of the arteries coming from this ventricle. If we want the fixative in the lungs, the fixative solution is introduced through the right ventricle. By perfusion, a single organ can be fixed if the fixative solution enters by the main artery that irrigates the whole organ. Fixation by perfusion is not always possible, like in many biopsies or in plants.

Fixation by perfusion is more effective than fixation by immersion because the fixative solution gets in contact with all cells of the perfused structure very quickly. In this way, the penetration speed of the fixative is not a limiting feature.

Before the introduction of the fixative in the vascular system, the blood should be removed with an oxygenated saline solution. Otherwise, the fixative may fix blood, coagulates it and produces thrombus. This may seal some parts of the vascular circuit that prevents the fixative solution entering some parts of the sample. As in the fixation by immersion, the pH and osmolarity of the fixative solution, and the fixation time, must be set properly.

Fixation by perfusion of a complete animal. The fixative solution is introduced through the vascular system. Pressure is provided by a peristaltic pump. The fixative solution enters via the left ventricle (lV) and reach the aorta. This artery and its branches distribute the fixative through the body (excepting the pulmonary circuit). The fixative arrives to and fills the capillary net, where most of the fixation process occurs. After that, fixative solution is gathered by venous system that converges in the right auricle (rA). This heart chamber is opened with a small cut to open the circuit and allow the fixative solution to leave the vascular system and the body. lA: left auricle; rV; right ventricle.

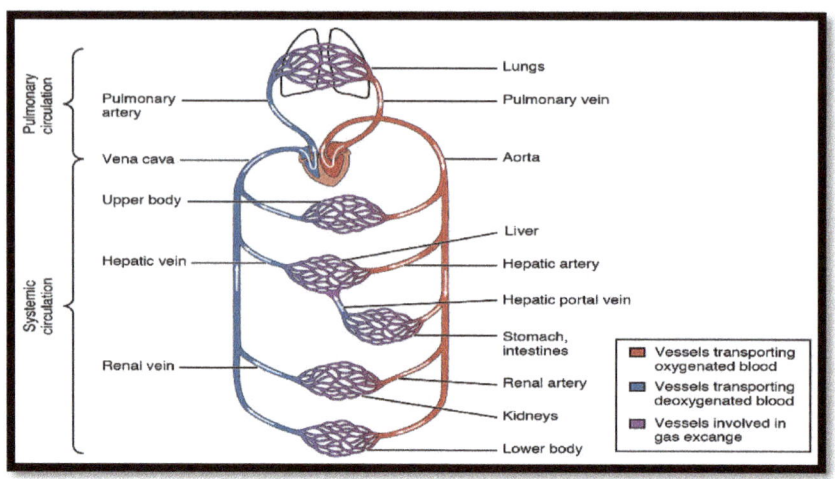

Fig. 2. Blood Flow Through the Heart

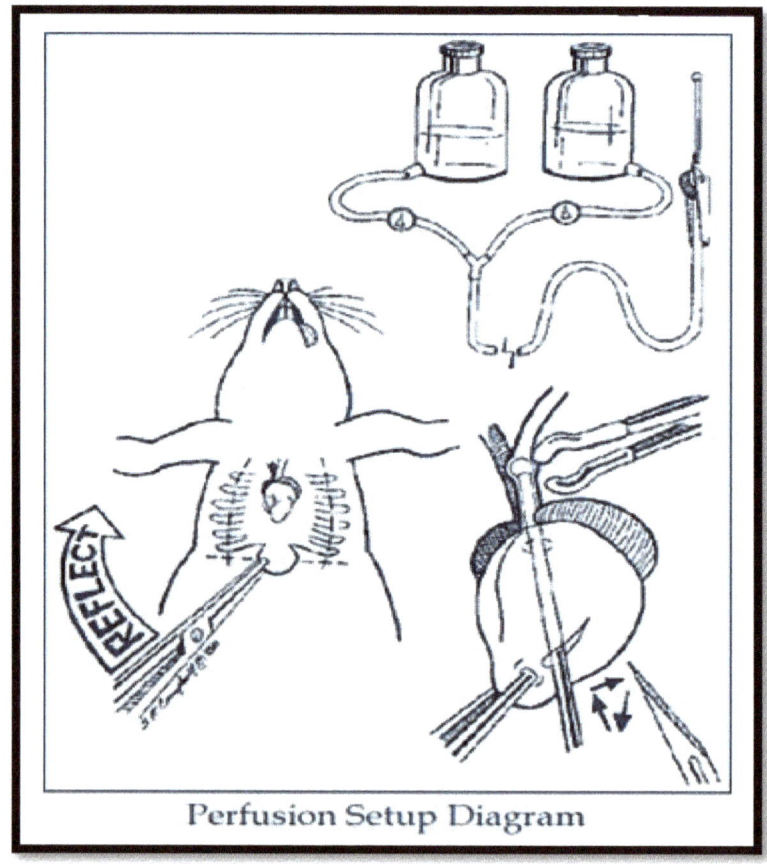

Fig. 3. Design of Perfusion set up

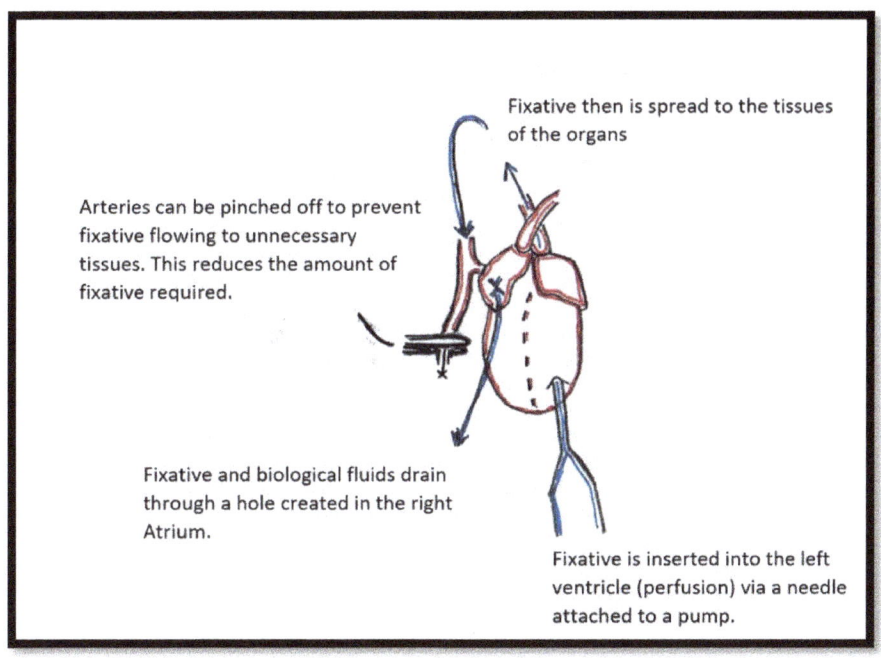

Fig. 4. Fixation of tissue through Perfusion set up.

Factors affecting fixation

Size and thickness of the piece of tissue

Tissue covered by mucous or blood may have slow penetration of fixative

Tissue containing fat is fixed slowly.

P^H-Satisfactory fixation occurs at P^H 6 to 8

Temperature – Usually at room temperature (for electron microscopy -0-4c)

Osmality of fixative – Fixative should be isotonic

Hypertonic solutions –Cell shrinkage

Hypotonic solution – Swelling cells & poor fixation.

Classification of fixatives into three main groups

Group A –

Microanatomical fixative

Cytological fixative

Histochemical fixative

Group B-
Coagulant fixatives
Non coagulant fixatives

Group C –
Simple
Aldehydes
Oxidizing agents
Protein denaturing agents
Unknown mechanism
Compound fixative

Group A (Based on structure to be preserved)

Micro anatomical fixative

They preserve anatomy of tissues and various layers of tissues in relation to each other
Formalin based fixative
Buffered Glutaraldehyde
Zenker fluid, Zenkers formal
Formal calcium

Fixatives are divided into three main groups

A. Microanatomical fixatives - such fixatives preserves the anatomy of the tissue.

B. Cytological fixatives - such fixation are used to preserve intracellular structures or inclusion.

C. Histochemical fixatives : Fixative used to preserve the chemical nature of the tissue for it to be demonstrated further. Freeze drying technique is best suited for this purpose.

Microanatomical fixatives

1. 10% (v/v) formalin in 0.9% sodium chloride (normal saline). This has been the routine fixative of choice for many years, but this has now been replaced by buffered formal or by formal calcium acetate

2. Buffered Formalin
(a) Formalin 10ml
(b) Acid sodium phosphate - 0.4 gm (monohydrate)
(c) Anhydrous disodium - 0.65 gm phosphate
(d) Water to 100 ml
- Best overall fixative

3. Formal calcium (Lillie : 1965)
(a) Formalin : 10 ml
(b) Calcium acetate 2.0 gm
(c) Water to 100 ml

• **Specific features**
- They have a near neutral pH
- Formalin pigment (acid formaldehyde haematin) is not formed

4. Buffered formal sucrose (Holt and Hicks, 1961)
(a) Formalin : 10ml
(b) Sucrose : 7.5 gm
(c) M/15 phosphate to 100 ml buffer (pH 7.4)

• **Specific features**
- This is an excellent fixative for the preservation of fine structure phospholipids and some enzymes.
- It is recommended for combined cytochemistry and electron microscopic studies.
- It should be used cold (4°C) on fresh tissue.

5. Alcoholic formalin
Formalin 10 ml
70-95% alcohol 90 ml

6. Acetic alcoholic formalin
Formalin 5.0ml
Glacial acetic acid 5.0 ml
Alcohol 70% 90.0 ml

7. Formalin ammonium bromide
Formalin 15.0 ml
Distilled water 85.0 ml
Ammonia bromide 2.0 gm

• **Specific features :** Preservation of neurological tissues especially when gold and silver impregnation is employed

8. Heidenhain Susa
(a) Mercuric chloride 4.5gm
(b) Sodium chloride 0.5 gm
(c) Trichloroacetic acid 2.0 gm
(d) Acetic acid 4.0 ml
(e) Distilled water to 100 ml

• **Specific features**
- Excellent fixative for routine biopsy work
- Allows brilliant staining with good cytological detail
- Gives rapid and even penetration with minimum shrinkage
- Tissue left in its for over 24 hours becomes bleached and excessively hardened.
- Tissue should be treated with iodine to remove mercury pigment

9. Zenker's fluid
(a) Mercuric chloride 5gm
(b) Potassium dichromate 2.5 gm
(c) Sodium sulphate 1.0 gm
(d) Distilled water to 100 ml
(e) Add immediately before use : Glacial acetic acid : 5 ml

- **Specific features**
- Good routine fixative
- Give fairly rapid and even penetration
- It is not stable after the addition of acetic acid hence acetic acid (or formalin) should be added just before use

Washing of tissue in running water is necessary to remove excess Dichromate

10. Zenker formal (Helly's fluid)
(a) Mercuric chloride - 5 gm
(b) Potassium dichromate 2.5 gm
(c) Sodium sulphate 1.0 gm
(d) Distilled water to 100 ml
(e) Add formalin immediately before use 5 ml

- **Specific features**
- It is excellent micro anatomical fixative
- Excellent fixative for bone marrow spleen and blood containing organs
- As with Zenker's fluid it is necessary to remove excess dichromate and mercuric pigment

11. B5 stock solution
Mercuric chloride 12 gm
Sodium acetate 2.5gm
Distilled water 200ml
B5 Working solution
B5 stock solution 20ml
Formalin (40% w/v formaldehyde) 2 ml

- **Specific Features**
- B5 is widely advocated for fixation of lymph node biopsies both to improve the cytological details and to enhance immunoreactivity.
ant immunoglobulin antiserum used in phenotyping of B cell neoplasm.
Procedure

_ Prepare working solution just before use
_ Fix small pieces of tissue (7x7x2.5mm) for 1-6 hours at room temperature
_ Process routinely to paraffin.

12. Bouin's fluid
(a) Saturated aqueous picric acid 75ml
(b) Formalin 25ml
(c) Glacial acetic acid 5 ml

• **Specific features**
- Penetrates rapidly and evenly and causes little shrinkage
- Excellent fixative for testicular and intestinal biopsies because it gives very good nuclear details, in testes is used for oligospermia and infertility studies
- Good fixative for glycogen
- It is necessary to remove excess picric acid by alcohol treatment

13. Gender's fluid - better fixative for glycogen.
(a) Saturated picric acid in 95% v/v/ alcohol 80ml
(b) Formalin 15ml
(c) Glacial acetic acid 5ml

Cytological fixatives
Subdivided into
(A) Nuclear fixatives
(B) Cytoplasmic fixatives

A. Nuclear fixatives :
As the name suggests it gives good nuclear fixation. This group includes

1. Carnoy's fluid.
(a) Absolute alcohol 60ml
(b) Chloroform 30ml
(c) Glacial acetic acid 10 ml

• **Specific features**
- It penetrates very rapidly and gives excellent nuclear fixation.
- Good fixative for carbohydrates.
- Nissl substance and glycogen are preserved.
- It causes considerable shrinkage.
- It dissolves most of the cytoplasmic elements. Fixation is usually complete in 1-2 hours.
For small pieces 2-3 mm thick only 15 minutes in needed for fixation.

2. Clarke's fluid
(a) Absolute alcohol 75 ml
(b) Glacial acetic acid 25 ml.

Specific features
- Rapid, good nuclear fixation and good preservation of cytoplasmic elements.
- It in excellent for smear or cover slip preparation of cell cultures or chromosomal analysis.

3. New Comer's fluid.
(a) Isopropranolol 60 ml
(b) Propionic acid 40ml
(c) Petroleum ether 10 ml.
(d) Acetone 10 ml.
(e) Dioxane 10 ml.

• **Specific features**
- Devised for fixation of chromosomes
- It fixes and preserves mucopolysacharides. Fixation in complete in 12-18 hours.

(b) Cytoplasmic Fixatives
(1) Champy's fluid
(a) 3g/dl Potassium dichromate 7ml.
(b) 1% (V/V) chromic acid 7 ml.
(c) 2gm/dl osmium tetraoxide 4 ml.

- **Specific features**
- This fixative cannot be kept hence prepared fresh.
- It preserves the mitochondrial fat and lipids.

Points to Remember
1. **10% buffered formalin** is the commonest fixative.
2. Tissues may be kept in 10% buffered formalin for long duration.
3. Volume of the fixative should be at least ten times of the volume of the specimen. The specimen should be completely submerged.
4. Special fixatives are used for preserving particular tissues.
5. **Formalin vapour**s cause throat/ eye irritation hence mask/ eye glasses and gloves should be used.
6. Tissues should be well fixed before dehydration.
7. Penetration of fixatives takes some time. It is necessary that the bigger specimen should be given cuts so that the central part does not remain unfixed.
8. **Mercury pigment must be removed with Lugol's iodine.**
9. Biopsies cannot be kept for more than 24 hours in bouin's fluid without changing the alcohol.
10. **Glutaraldehyde and osmium tetra oxide** are used as fixatives for electron microscopy.

STAINING TECHNIQUES

Introduction

Histology means the science of the tissues.

histos is Greek for web or tissue

logia is Greek for branch of learning

Tissue was first used to describe the different textures of body parts being dissected by an anatomist.

What kinds of histological stains are there?

Most cells are colourless and transparent, and therefore histological sections have to be stained in some way to make the cells visible. The techniques used can either be non-specific, staining most of the cells in much the same way, or specific, selectively staining particular chemical groupings or molecules within cells or tissues. Staining usually works by using a dye, that stains some of the cells components a bright colour, together with a counterstain that stains the rest of the cell a different colour.

Basophilic and acidophilic staining.

Acidic dyes react with cationic or basic components in cells. Proteins and other components in the cytoplasm are basic, and will bind to acidic dyes.

Another way of saying this is that cytoplasmic proteins are acidophilic (acid liking - i.e. bind to acidic dyes).

Basic dyes react with anionic or acidic components in cells. Nucleic acids are acidic, and therefore bind to basic dyes. Another way of saying this is that nucleic acids are basophilic (basic liking).

What is H&E ?

The most commonly used staining system is called H&E (Haemotoxylin and Eosin). H&E contains the two dyes haemotoxylin and eosin.

Eosin is an acidic dye: it is negatively charged (general formula for acidic dyes is: Na^+dye^-). It stains basic (or acidophilic) structures red or pink. This is also sometimes termed 'eosinophilic'.

Thus the cytoplasm is stained pink in the picture below, by H&E staining.

Haematoxylin can be considered as a basic dye (general formula for basic dyes is: $dye^+ Cl^-$). Haematoxylin is actually a dye called hematein (obtained from the log-wood tree) used in combination with aluminium ions (Al^{3+}). It is used to stain acidic (or basophilic) structures a purplish blue. (Haematoxylin is not strictly a basic dye, but it is used with a 'mordant' that makes this stain act as a basic dye. The mordant (aluminium salts) binds to the tissue, and then haematoxylin binds to the mordant, forming a tissue-mordant-haematoxylin linkage.)

Thus the nucleus is stained purple in the picture below, by H&E staining.

This means that the nucleus, and parts of the cytoplasm that contain RNA stain up in one colour (purple), and the rest of the cytoplasm stains up a different colour (pink).

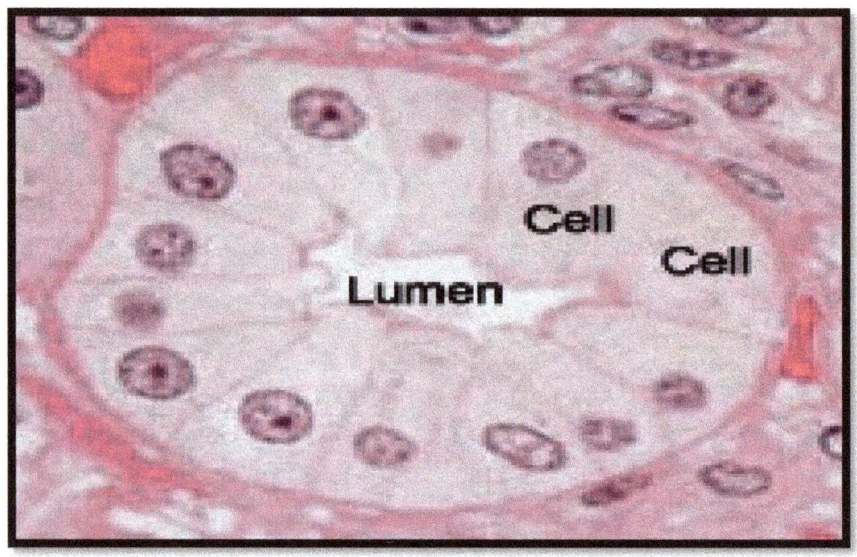

Fig. 5. Figure depicts a group of cells lining a duct. Nuclei are distinct with nucleoli.

What structures are stained purple (basophilic)?

DNA (heterochromatin and the nucleolus) in the nucleus, and RNA in ribosomes and in the rough endoplasmic reticulum are both acidic, and so haemotoxylin binds to them and stains them purple. Some extracellular materials (i.e. carbohydrates in cartilage) are also basophilic.

What structures are stained pink (eosinophilic or acidophilic)?

Most proteins in the cytoplasm are basic, and so eosin binds to these proteins and stains them pink. This includes cytoplasmic filaments in muscle cells, intracellular membranes, and extracellular fibres.

Principle

Hematoxylin is extracted from **Hematoxylon campechianum** tree upon which on oxidation, hematein is produced from hematoxylin, the dye used in the hematoxylin and Eosin staining technique. Adding a mordant enables hematein to bind to the anionic elements of the tissues. Hematoxylin without eosin acts a counterstain in immunohistochemical and hybridization protocols that use colorimetric substrates (such as alkaline phosphatase or peroxidase)

Eosin dye is acidic dye hence it as a negative charge (eosinophilic). Therefore it stains the basic structures of a cell (acidophils), giving them a red or pink color, for example, the cytoplasm is positively charged, and therefore it will take up the eosin dye, and appear pink.

Hematoxylin dyes are basic dyes, hence they are positively charged. Therefore it will stain the acidic structures of tissues and cell structures (basophilic), purplish-blue. Hematoxylin is not basic by itself. It has to be conjugated with a mordant (aluminum salt) before it is used so as to strengthen its positive charge for efficiency in binding to the tissue components. The mordant, which also defines the color of the stain, will bind to the tissue, then the hematoxylin will bind to the mordant to form a tissue-mordant-hematoxylin complex link. This will stain the nuclei and chromatin bodies purple.

H &E stain can be classified into three types: progressive, modified progressive, and regressive. Progressive staining takes place without a differentiator for removing any excess dye after adding hematoxylin. This cause background staining to occur in charged slides. Its mainly used to stain Mucin. While the Modified progressive and regressive, use a differentiator in removing excessive dyes. It is used for the demonstration of nucleus content.

Hematoxylin and Eosin (H&E) Staining – Manual Protocol (From Baylor College of Medicine) Protocol for H&E staining:

- Place slides containing paraffin sections in a slide holder (glass or metal)
- Deparaffinize and rehydrate sections:

3 x 3′ Xylene (blot excess xylene before going into ethanol)

3 x 3′ 100% ethanol 1 x 3′ 95% ethanol

1 x 3′ 80% ethanol

1 x 5′ deionized H2O

- While sections are in water, skim surface of hematoxalin with a Kimwipe to remove oxidized particles. Blot excess water from slide holder before going into hematoxalin.

- Hematoxalin staining:

1 x 3′ Hematoxalin Rinse deionized water

1 x 5′ Tap water (to allow stain to develop)

Dip 8-12x (fast) Acid ethanol (to destain)

Rinse 2 x 1′ Tap water

Rinse 1 x 2′ Deionized water (can leave overnight at this stage)

(Blot excess water from slide holder before going into eosin)

Eosin staining and dehydration:

1 x 30 sec Eosin (up to 45 seconds for an older batch of eosin)

3 x 5′ 95% ethanol

3 x 5′ 100% ethanol (blot excess ethanol before going into xylene)

3 x 15′ Xylene

- Coverslip slides using Permount (xylene based).
- Place a drop of Permount on the slide using a glass rod, taking care to leave no bubbles.
- Angle the coverslip and let fall gently onto the slide. Allow the Permount to spread beneath the coverslip, covering all the tissue.
- Dry overnight in the hood.

Reagents for H&E staining:

- Acid Ethanol: 1 ml concentrated HCl + 400 ml 70% ethanol
- Hematoxylin: Poly Scientific (Bayshore, NY) #s212A Harris hematoxylin with glacial acetic acid
- Eosin: Poly Scientific (Bayshore, NY) #s176 Eosin Phloxine stain, working
- Permount: Fisher Scientific #SP15-100 Histological mounting medium

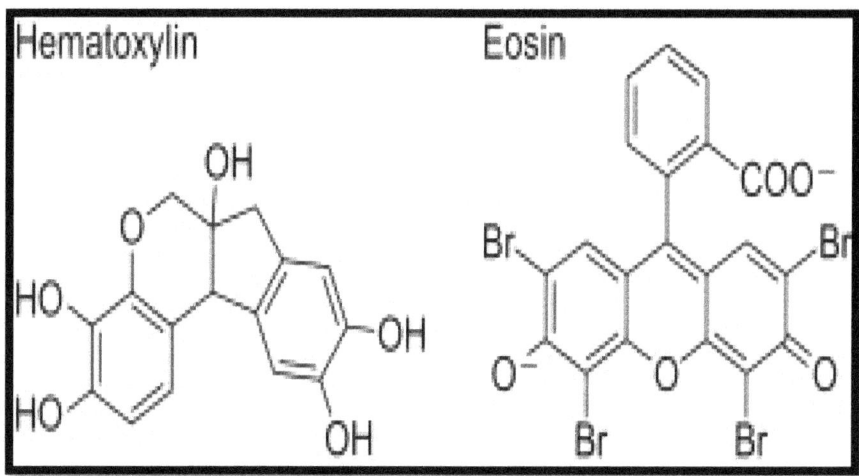

Fig. 6. The structures of hematoxylin and eosin. The structures of hematoxylin (which binds avidly and rapidly to nucleic acids) and eosin (which binds avidly and rapidly to proteins) is presented. The signal from each stain, unlike the precipitates from DAB and NBT/BCIP, are easily removed from the cells and will not interfere with in situ hybridization or immunohistochemistry.

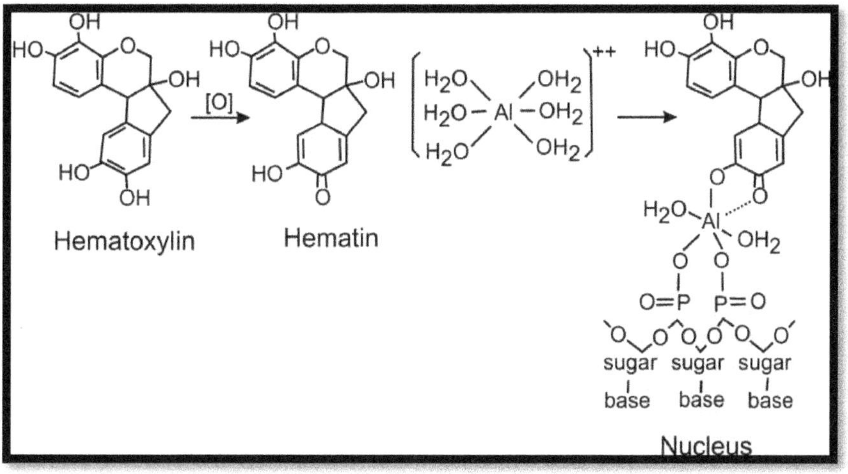

Fig. 7. Mechanism of reaction of nucleus with haematoxylin.

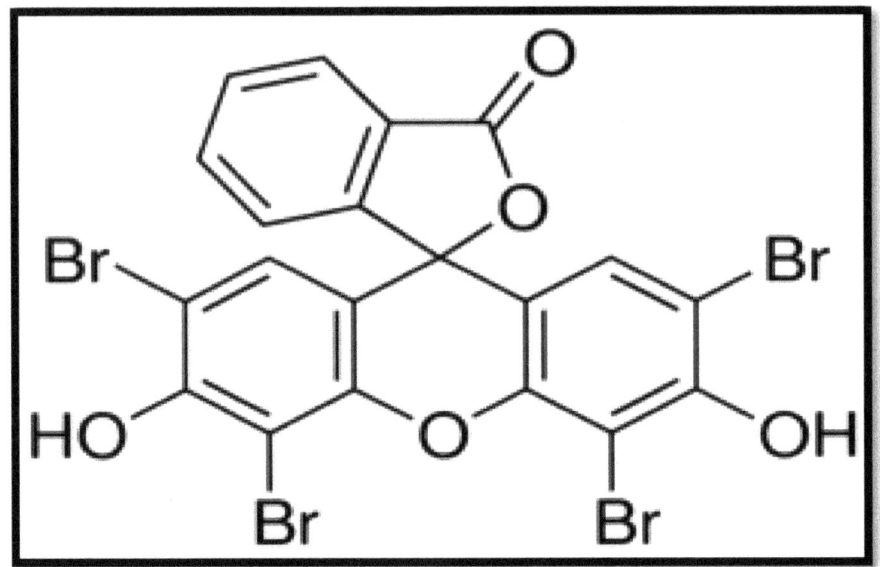

Fig. 8. Structure of Eosin Y

Eosin Y sodium salt

Alternate Names: 2',4',5',7'-Tetrabromofluorescein; Acid Red 87

Application: Eosin Y sodium salt is a red fluorescent dye from the xanthene family

Molecular Weight: 691.85

Molecular Formula: $C_{20}H_6Br_4O_5 \cdot 2Na$

Dye content ~99 %

Types of Eosin

Eosin is any one of a class of rose-colored stains or dyes and many types can be obtained commercially. Some of the more common ones are:

Eosin

Eosin Y (most widely used and is soluble in both alcohol and water)

Alcoholic eosin Y

Eosin B

Eosin- phloxine

Picro-eosin

What are the uses of Hematoxylin & Eosin Stain ?

Hematoxylin & Eosin is the most widely used stain in medical diagnosis and is often the gold standard.

As an example, when a pathologist looks at a biopsy of a suspected cancer, with Hematoxylin & Eosin.

Result of Hematoxylin & Eosin Stain

Nuclei , Calcium salts ,urates & Bacteria – stain in blue color

Also Cytoplasm, Connective tissues , erythrocytes – stain in shaded pink color.

Advantages of Hematoxylin & Eosin Staining

1. Provide excellent nuclear details – Outline , chromatin pattern & nucleoli
2. Provide Important information helpful for diagnosis – keratinization , oncocytes & psammoma bodies
3. Not very expensive stain
4. Can be used to diagnose a wide-range of histopathologic conditions.

Disadvantages of Hematoxylin & Eosin Staining

1. Long staining time
2. H&E staining does not always provide enough contrast to differentiate all tissues & cellular structures

Stages of staining the tissues with H & E Method

Xylene	5 minutes
Xylene	2 minutes
100% ethanol	2 minutes
100% ethanol	2 minutes
95% ethanol	2 minutes
70% ethanol	2 minutes
Water wash	2 minutes

Hematoxylin	1-2 minutes
Water wash	1 minute
Differentiator (mild acid)	1 minute
Water wash	1 minute
Bluing	1 minute
Water wash	1 minute
70% ethanol	2 minutes
90% ethanol	4-5 minutes
95% ethanol	2 minutes
Eosin	1-2 minutes
95% ethanol	1 minute
100% ethanol	2 minutes
100 % ethanol	2 minutes
100% ethanol	2 minute
Xylene	2 minutes
Xylene	2 minutes
Coverslip	

1. Hematoxylin Harris

Hematoxylin 5.0 g

Ammonium/ Potassium Alum 100 g

Mercuric Oxide 2.5 g

Alcohol 95% 50 mL

Distilled Water 1000 mL

Appearance : Maroon purplish solution.

2. Eosin (AQU.)

2% Eosin-Y 2.0 g
Distilled water 100 mL

Appearance: Dark reddish solution.

ELECTRON MICROSCOPY PROCEDURES MANUAL

SPECIMEN PREPARATION PROTOCOL TEM

1. FIXATION:

Tissue can be fixed by immersion or perfusion. The most commonly used method is immersion. Fixation time is variable, depending on tissue, but usually from 4 hours to overnight at 4 degrees (refrigerator).

a. Primary Fixative:

 1/2 strength Karnovsky's.

- 2% Paraformaldehyde/2.5% Glutaraldehyde
- This is buffered with a 0.2M Cacodylate Buffer

Note: Always use the fixative in the fume hood and wear gloves. Glutaraldehyde fixes skin and cacodylate buffer contains arsenic.

b. 0.1M Cacodylate Buffer wash

c. Post Fixative: 2% aqueous OsO4/0.2 M Cacodylate Buffer

- A 1:1 solution for 2 hours in the refrigerator

d. 0.1 M Cacodylate Buffer wash

2. DEHYDRATION:

 Dehydration with ethanol:
35% ETOH 15 min. and decant (optional)
50% ETOH 15 min. and decant
70% ETOH 15 min. and decant
 95% ETOH 15 min. and decant
100%ETOH 15 min. and decant
100% ETOH 15 min. and decant
Propylene Oxide 15 min. and decant

Propylene Oxide 15 min. and decant

1:1 PO/Epon resin overnight

- The dehydrating times should be adjusted to size and kind of tissue.
- The resin is an Epon 812 recipe .

3. EMBEDDING:

Embedding with Epon:

- Next morning, change out to fresh Epon 812 for 1-3 hours.
- Embed (always) in fresh Epon 812
- Polyethylene capsules are placed in a holder and numbered strips of paper are inserted.

A drop of fresh Epon 812 is placed in the capsules and the specimen is transferred to the appropriate capsule.

- The "blocks" are cured for 48 hours in a 60 degree oven.

Procedure

The embedding medium is prepared by gravimetrically adding the components singly into a flask. The composition which is recommended is as follows:

Ingredients	Mass (g)
Vinylcyclohexene dioxide	10
Diglycidyl ether of Polyproplyeneglycol D.E.R. 736	6.3
Nonenyl succinic anhydride	26
Dimethylaminoethanol D.M.A.E.	0.4

N.B.

DO NOT STIR VIGOROUSLY (use stir magnet)

Variations in these compositions can be obtained from reference below. Exact weight should be used for optimum performance. It is generally desirable to add the dimethylaminoethanol catalyst last after gentle mixing of the previous components. Should bubbles form, they may be drawn off with a gentle vacuum applied to the mixing container.

4. SECTIONING:

- 1 micron or thick sections are taken to find the area of interest
- Take ultra thin sections (~70nm) and place on grids

5. POST STAINING:

- Stain grids in uranyl acetate for 2 hrs.
- Stain grids in lead citrate for 5 min.

** This procedure is the basic TEM procedure.

N.B.: Each and every sample that comes to us is evaluated and the procedure is adjusted to make sure the best results will be obtained.

Safety notes: Glutaraldehyde and osmium tetroxide fix cells by cross-linking their proteins via the amine groups (glutaraldehyde) or their phospholipids (osmium). They are harmful to living cells and you should avoid exposure to them. I prefer to use them in a fume hood. Fixatives are volatile and can fix any cells they contact - other cells in the lab or in respiratory epithelium, corneas, epithelial cells on your hand, etc. The good thing is that the fixatives cannot penetrate tissue more than a millimeter or two, so exposure to them rarely causes any permanent damage.

The plastics used to embed the tissue are more dangerous than the fixatives and many of the components of the plastic have been shown to cause cancer in rats or mice. During the embedding process the plastics are dissolved in solvent that can easily carry the plastic into your tissues and through any plastic gloves you may wear. In contrast to fixatives, whose actions are immediate and apparent, the consequences of exposure to the plastic resins are not apparent for years. Please be careful with the plastic resins prior to polymerization into hard blocks. Plastic-containing waste solutions should be kept in a container in the EM lab.

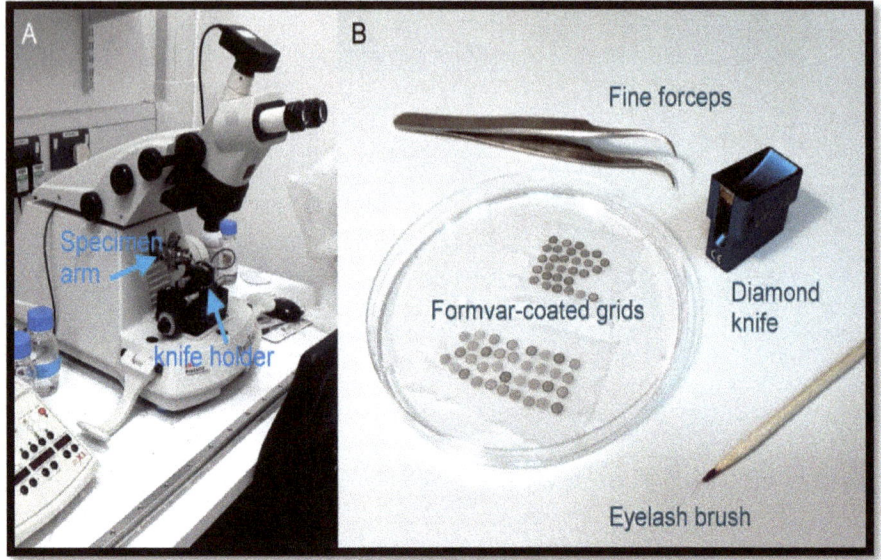

Fig. 9. Equipment needed for ultramicrotomy. **(A) ultramicrotome; (B) knife, forceps, grids, and eyelash brush.**

Trimming the Block

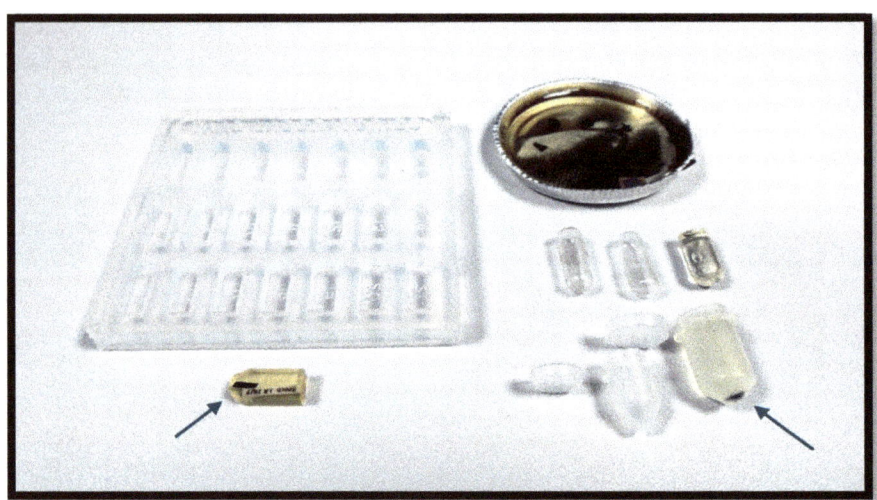

Fig. 10. **Different types of embedding moulds and capsules.** Arrows indicate the sample in the resin blocks.

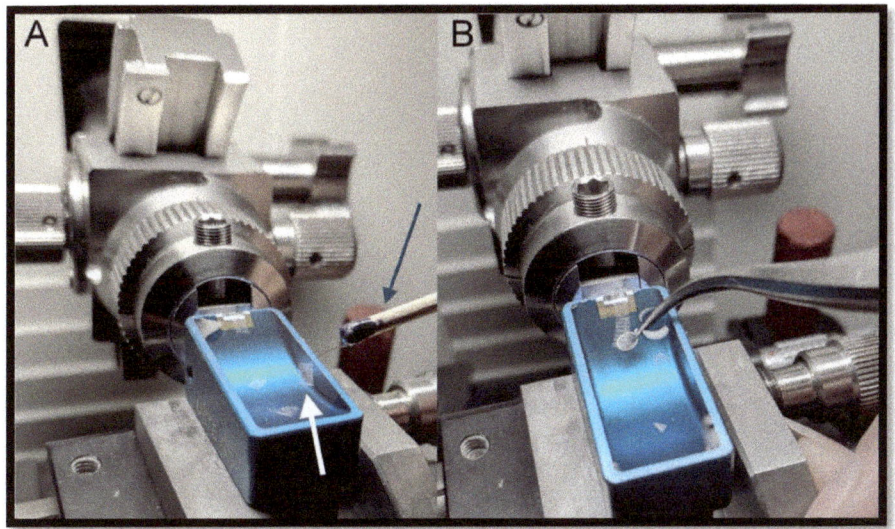

Fig. 11. **Manipulation of sections.** Sections (white arrow) being manipulated with an eyelash brush (blue arrow) (A). The sections are then collected onto a grid (B).

CHAPTER II

ANATOMICAL POSITION, HISTOLOGICAL AND ULTRA STRUCTURAL OBSERVATION OF SOME IMPORTANT ENDOCRINE GLANDS

IMPORTANT ENDOCRINE GLANDS

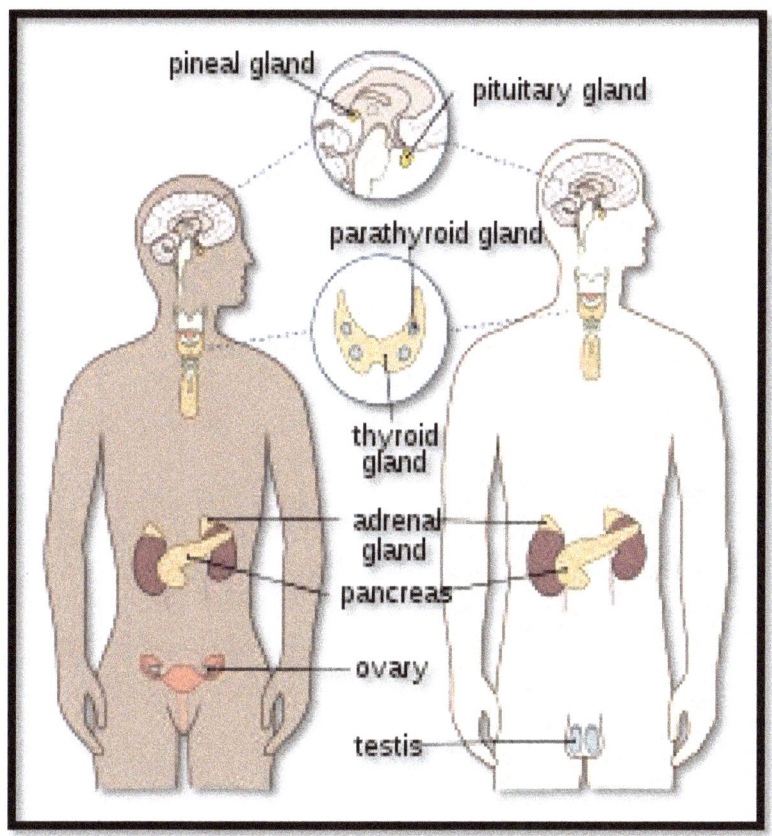

Fig. 12. Important endocrine glands are marked within the figure.

Hypothalamus: It controls the body temperature, regulates emotions, hunger, thirst, sleep, moods and allow the production of hormones.

Pineal: Pineal is also known as the thalamus. It produces serotonin derivatives of melatonin, which affects sleep patterns.

Parathyroid: This gland helps in controlling the amount of calcium present in the body.

Thymus: It helps in the production of T-cells, functioning of the adaptive immune system and maturity of the thymus.

Thyroid: It produces hormones that affect the heart rate and how calories are burnt.

Adrenal: This gland produces the hormones that control the sex drive, cortisol and stress hormone.

Pituitary: It is also termed as the "master control gland,". This is because the pituitary gland helps in controlling other glands. Moreover, it develops the hormones that trigger growth and development.

Pancreas: This gland is involved in the production of insulin hormones, which plays a crucial role in maintaining blood sugar levels.

Testes: In men, the testes secrete the male sex hormone, testosterone. It also produces sperm.

Ovaries: In the female reproductive system, the ovaries release estrogen, progesterone, testosterone and other female sex hormones.

LIST OF IMPORTANT HORMONES

Cortisol – It has been named as the "stress hormone" as it helps the body in responding to stress. This is done by increasing the heart rate, elevating blood sugar levels etc.

Estrogen-This is the main sex hormone present in women which bring about puberty, prepares the uterus and body for pregnancy and even regulates the menstrual cycle. Estrogen level changes during menopause because of which women experience many uncomfortable symptoms.

Melatonin – It primarily controls the circadian rhythm or sleep cycles.

Progesterone – It is a female sex hormone also responsible for menstrual cycle, pregnancy and embryogenesis.

Testosterone – This is the most important sex hormone synthesized in men, which cause puberty, muscle mass growth, and strengthen the bones and muscles, increase bone density and controls facial hair growth.

ADRENAL GLAND (SUPRA RENAL GLAND)

Anatomical Position

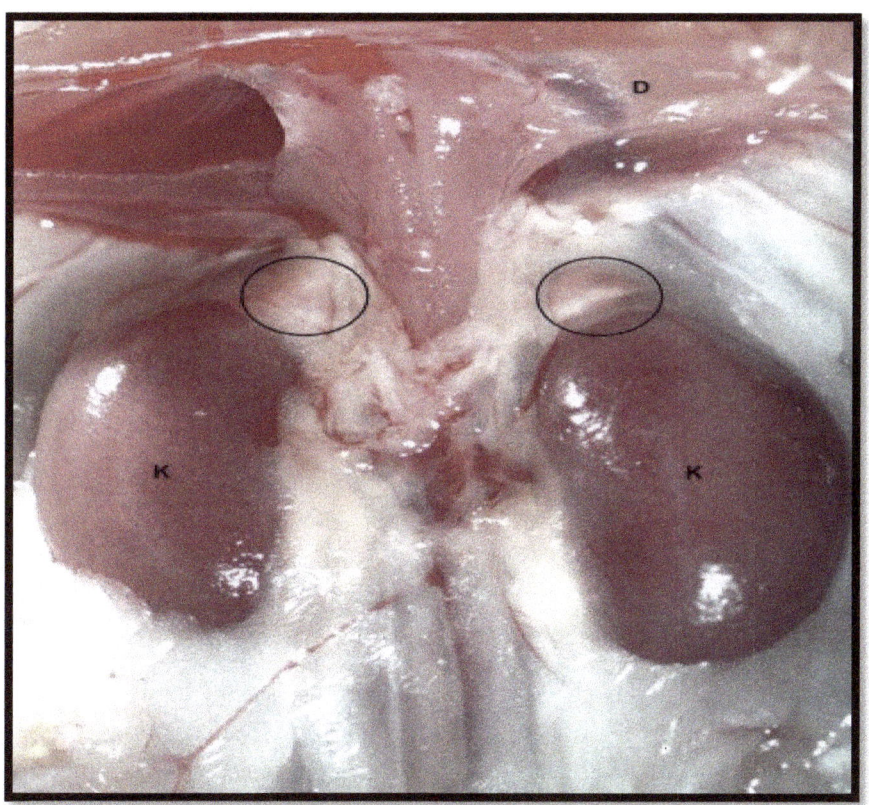

Fig. 13. Exact location of the suprarenal gland / adrenal gland

Location of Adrenal Cortex

The adrenal glands are a pair of triangular or round bodies located adjacent to the superior pole of each kidney. They show a combined weight of about 10–15 g in humans, and 40–60 mg in rats. Each Adrenal gland has an outer cortex which produces steroid hormones and an inner medulla which is called Adrenal Cortex.

Structure of Adrenal Cortex

Each adrenal gland is enclosed in a connective tissue capsule and consists of two functionally distinct parts: a superficial yellowish part called Adrenal cortex, and a deeper brownish part known as adrenal medulla. The volume of the cortex is about ten times the medulla. The adrenal cortex secretes steroid hormones called adreno-corticosteroids or corticoids, while the medulla secretes catecholamines.

Histology of Adrenal Cortex

The adrenal cortex histologically comprises of the following three zones:

1. Zona glomerulosa
2. Zona fasciculata
3. Zona reticularis

Function of the Adrenal Cortex

The adrenal cortex produces a handful of hormones necessary for fluid and electrolyte (salt) balance in the body such as cortisol and aldosterone. The adrenal cortex also makes small amounts of sex hormones but this only becomes important if overproduction is present (most sex hormones are produced by the testes and ovaries).

Histological Structures of the Adrenal Gland

The adrenal gland consists of two ontogenetically, structurally and functionally distinct endocrine tissues, the cortex and the medulla. The cortex is mesodermal in origin and derived from proliferation of the coelomic epithelium. The medulla, on the other hand, is ectodermal in origin and neural crest-derived. It secretes catecholamines, i.e., adrenaline and noradrenaline, that facilitate the acute mammalian stress or "fight-or-flight" response.

Division of adrenal cortex

The cortex is further subdivided into concentric zones, the zona glomerulosa (zG), the zona fasciculata (zF) and the zona reticularis (zR), which were originally named by Arnold in 1866 from the morphological appearance or shape of the cells in each zone (glomus, ball ; fascis, bundle; and rete, net) rather than from function. Later it was established that each zone has specific endocrine functions.

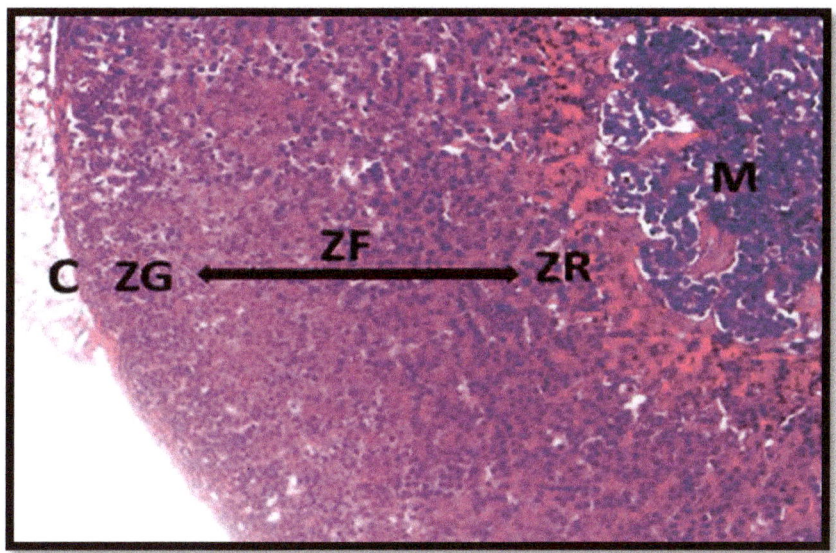

Fig. 14. Portion of the adrenal structures of rat (Histological , **H& E preparation**)
C : capsule ; ZG : zona glomerulosa ; ZF : zona fasciculata , ZR : zona reticularis

Zona glomerulosa

The outer zone is the zona glomerulosa and is composed of a thin region of columnar cells arranged in an arched or arcuate pattern. This zone is also called the zona multiformis in animals because of its different patterns of arrangement of secretory cells. The zona glomerulosa produces the steroid hormone aldosterone, which is responsible for increasing sodium reabsorption and stimulating potassium excretion by the kidneys and thereby indirectly regulating extracellular ☐fluid volume.

Zona fasciculata

The zona fas- ciculata is the thickest zone (70% of the cortex) and is composed of columns of secretory cells separated by prominent capillaries. The cells are polyhedral and have many intracellular lipid droplets. This zone produces glu- cocorticoids.

Zona reticularis

The zona reticularis is also composed of polyhedral cells, whose arrangement is less linear and more as round nests or clumps of cells. The zona reti- cularis produces glucocorticoids and in some species small amounts of sex steroids, namely, androgens, estro- gens, and progestins. This zone is more distinct in rats compared to mice.

Adrenal medulla

The cells of the adrenal medulla are derived from the neural crest. The secretory cells of the adrenal medulla are called chromaffin cells because of the formation of colored polymers of catecholamines after exposure to oxidizing agents, such as chromate. They secrete epinephrine or norepinephrine into the blood in response to acetylcholine or calcium ion. There are 3 types of adrenal medullary cells in adults: epinephrine cells (66– 75%), norepinephrine cells (25– 33%), and small granule-containing cells (SGC, 4% in mice and 1% in rats). The medullary cells produce other peptides in addition to epi- nephrine and norepinephrine, such as met-enkephalin, substance P, neurotensin, neuropeptide Y, and chromogranin A. In addition, the adrenal medulla contains pre- synaptic sympathetic ganglion cells.

Hormones secreted by the adrenal medulla are:

Epinephrine: Most people know epinephrine by its other name—adrenaline. This hormone rapidly responds to stress by increasing your heart rate and rushing blood to the muscles and brain. It also spikes your blood sugar level by helping convert glycogen to glucose in the liver. (Glycogen is the liver's storage form of glucose.)

Norepinephrine: Also known as noradrenaline, this hormone works with epinephrine in responding to stress. However, it can cause vasoconstriction (the narrowing of blood vessels). This results in high blood pressure.

ADRENAL GLAND ULTRASTRUCTURE

ULTRASTRUCTURAL DETAILS

Zona Glomerulosa region

The cells of ZG were arranged in arches just beneath the connective tissue capsule. They were recognized by their **euchromatic** nuclei. Their cytoplasm showed many **lipid** droplets. The mitochondria exhibited **shelf like** cristae .

Zona fasciculata region

In the ZF, the cells revealed **rounded euchromatic nuclei** and many **lipid droplets**. Numerous **mitochondria** with **vesicular cristae,** profiles of **smooth endoplasmic reticulum** and a small **Golgi complex** were further encountered .

Zona reticularis region

The cells of the ZR revealed abundant **mitochondria**. They were mainly rounded or ovoid in shape, variable in sizes with **vesicular or tubulo-vesicular** cristae and occupied most of the cytoplasm. Occasionally **lysosomes** and **lipofuscin** pigments were also seen. The cells further revealed well developed intercellular junctions .

Structure of Zona Glomerulosa region (Ultrastructure)

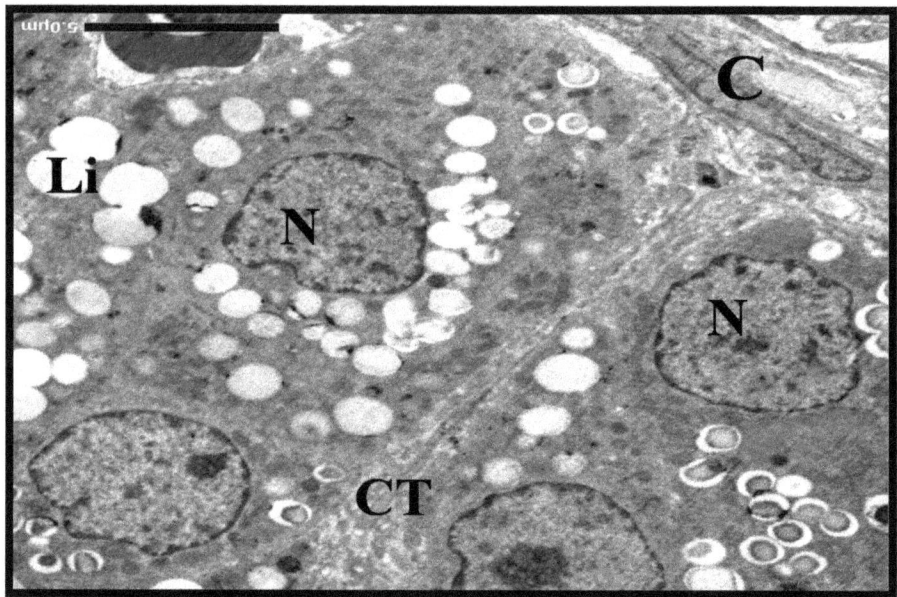

Fig. 15. **Electron micrographs of the adrenal cortex (a small portion) of rat showing a group of ZG** cells. Cells areseparated by thin connective tissue septa (CT). The connective tissue capsule (C) is seen overlying group of glomerulosa cells . The cells have euchromatic nuclei (N). The cytoplasm contains some lipid droplets (Li). c) A high magnification and mitochondria (M) with shelf like cristae in the cytoplasm. Li; lipid droplet, N; nucleus. x1500 .

Zona Fasciculata Region (Ultrastructure)

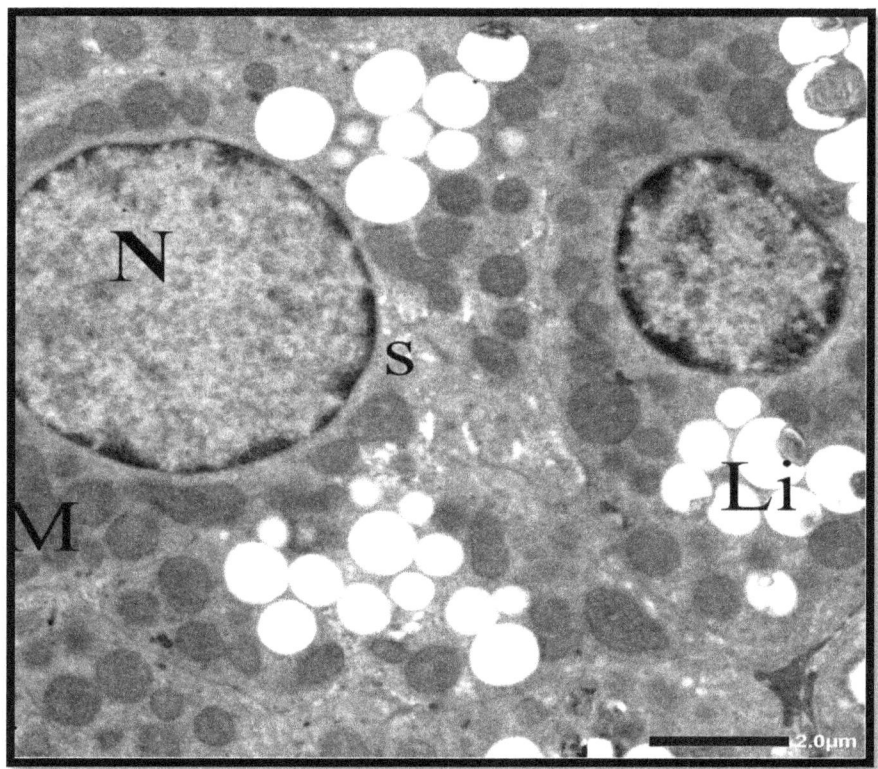

Fig. 16. **Electron micrographs of the zona fasciculata cells showing**; a) Adjacent cells with rounded euchromatic nuclei (N) and intracellular lipid droplets (Li) of varying sizes. The cytoplasm shows profiles of smooth endoplasmic reticulum (S). M; mitochondria. b) Parts of two adjacent fasciculata cells showing rounded mitochondria (M) with vesicular cristae and a small Golgi complex (G) . x2500.

Zona reticularis region (Ultrastructure)

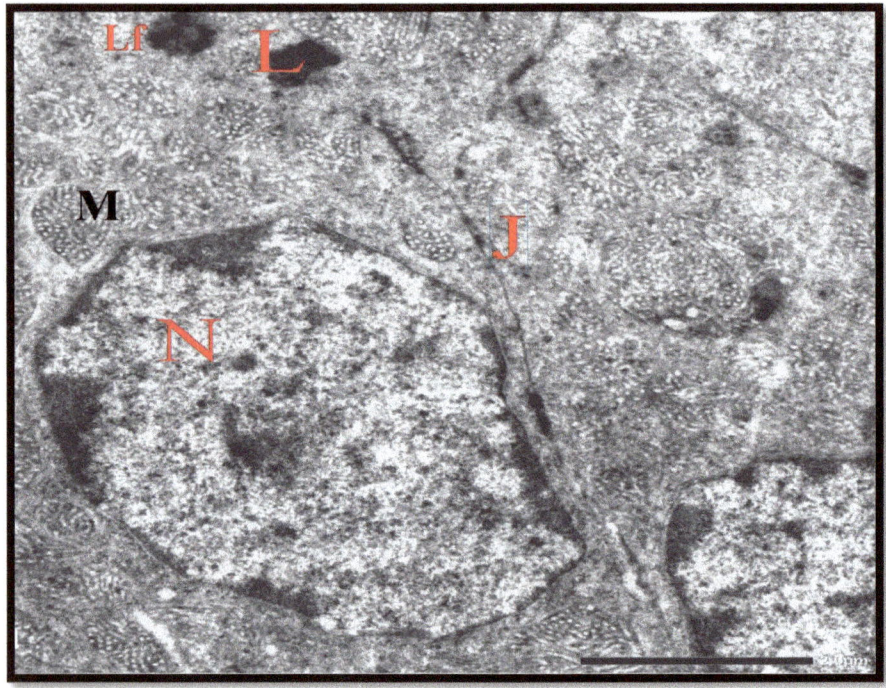

Fig.17. **Electron micrographs of ZR cells of the control group.** The cytoplasm shows numerous closely packed mitochondria (M), with tubulo-vesicular cristae. Lf; lipofuscin pigment in a, L; lysosome, J; desmosome junction, N; nucleus. x4000.

CONTRIBUTION OF SCIENTISTS – ON ADRENAL FUNCTION

A. Edward Calvin Kendall

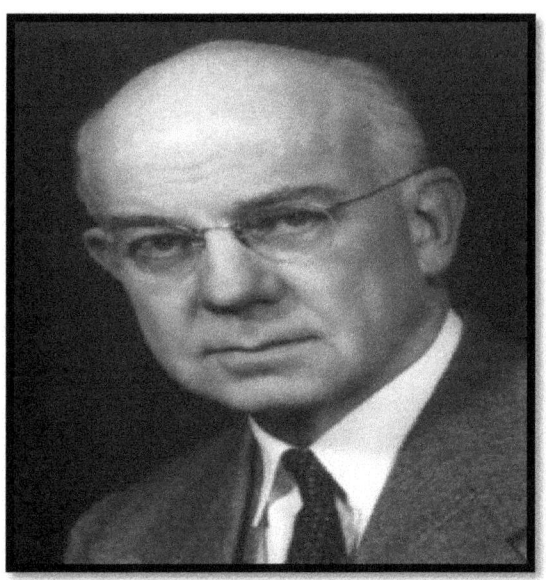

Edward Calvin Kendall

The Nobel Prize in Physiology or Medicine , 1950
Born: 8 March 1886, South Norwalk, **CT, USA**
Died: 4 May 1972, Princeton, **NJ, USA**
Affiliation at the time of the award: Mayo Clinic, Rochester, MN, USA
The Development of Cortisone as a Therapeutic Agent

Contribution

Kendall made several notable contributions to biochemistry and medicine. His most notable discovery was the isolation of thyroxine, although it was not the work he received the most accolades for. Along with associates, Kendall was involved with the isolation of glutathione and determining its structure. He also isolated several steroids from the adrenal gland cortex, one of which was initially called Compound E. Working with Mayo Clinic physician Philip Showalter Hench, Compound E was used to treat rheumatoid arthritis. The compound was eventually named cortisone. In 1950, Kendall and Hench, along with Swiss chemist Tadeus Reichstein were awarded the 1950 Nobel Prize in Physiology or Medicine for "their discoveries relating to the hormones of the adrenal cortex, their structure and biological effects.

B. Tadeus Reichstein

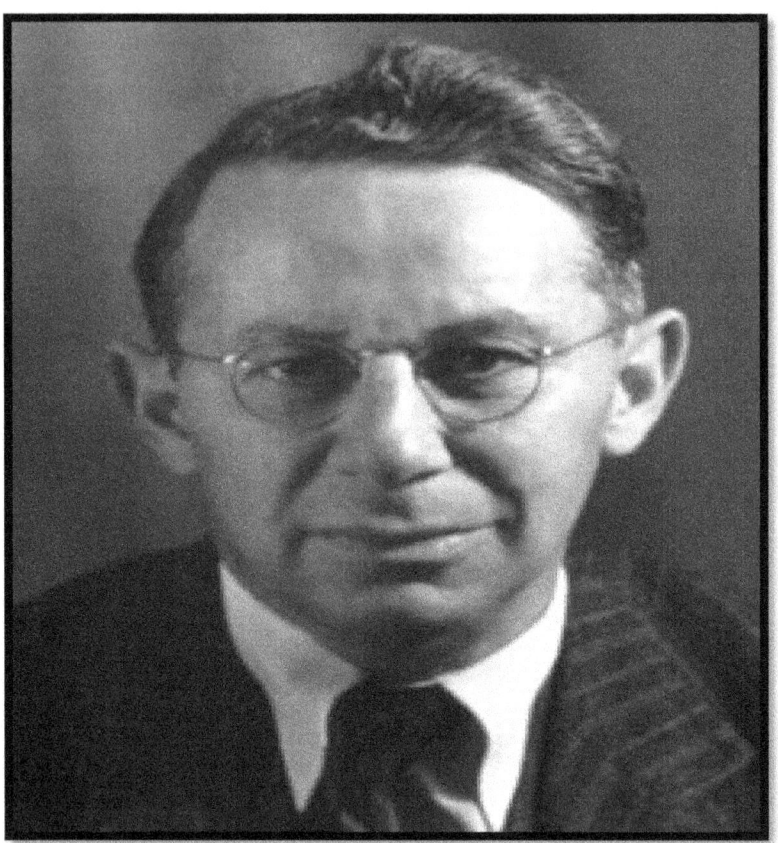

Tadeus Reichstein
The Nobel Prize in Physiology or Medicine 1950
Born: 20 July 1897, Wloclawek, Poland
Died: 1 August 1996, Basel, Switzerland
Affiliation at the time of the award: Basel University, Basel, Switzerland

Contribution

Reichstein was amongst the leading scientists in organic chemistry in the twentieth century. With his synthesis of Vitamin C by using microorganisms he combined chemical and biological methods, and thus introduced patterns that became standard in modern biotechnology. In 1950 he received the Nobel Prize for the discovery of the chemical structure of the corticosteroids, opening up an avenue leading to the uses of cortisone and other hormones as pharmaceuticals.

C. Philip Showalter Hench

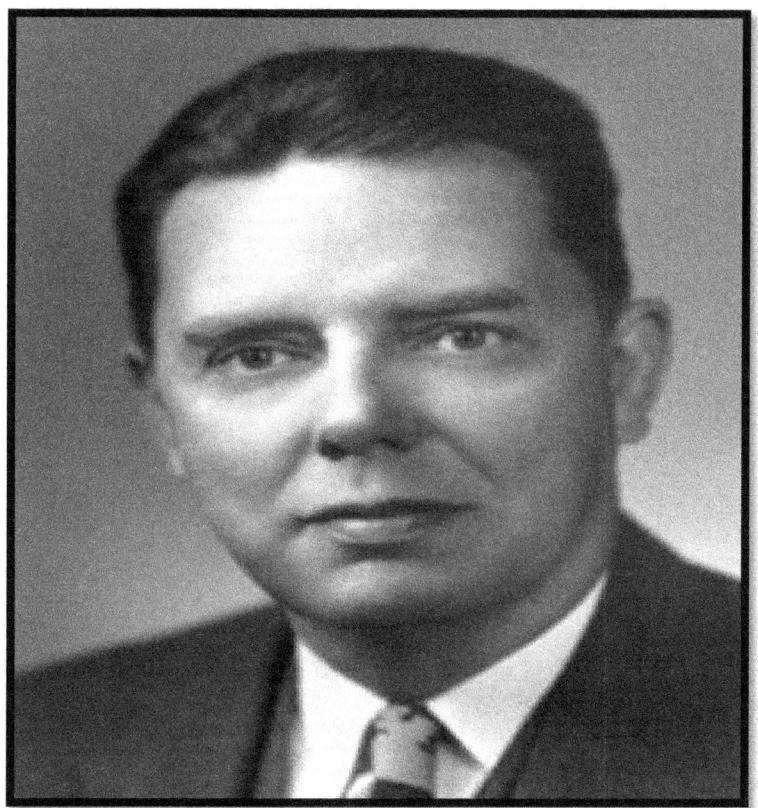

Philip Showalter Hench

The Nobel Prize in Physiology or Medicine 1950
Born: 28 February 1896, Pittsburgh, PA, USA
Died: 30 March 1965, Ocho Rios, Jamaica
Affiliation at the time of the award: Mayo Clinic, Rochester, MN, USA

Contribution

American physician who is known for his contribution in the treatment of rheumatism, an umbrella term that includes arthritis and other pains associated with the joints and muscles. His research with arthritis led him to discover that in some cases the symptoms can be reversed. He also successfully used cortisone and extracts of the pituitary and adrenal cortex to combat arthritis. He shared the Nobel Prize for physiology or medicine with E. C. Kendall and Tadeus Reichstein in 1950.

ADRENAL MEDULLA

Histology

The adrenal medulla occupies the central portion of the adrenal gland. This region of the adrenal glands contains basophilic staining cells, with a granular cytoplasm and no stored lipid. Adrenomedullary cells are called chromaffin cells (they stain brown with chromium salts). Chromaffin cells differentiate in the center of the adrenal gland in response to cortisol; some chromaffin cells also migrate to form paraganglia. The largest cluster of chromaffin cells outside the adrenal medulla is near the level of the inferior mesenteric artery and is referred to as the organ of Zuckerkandl.

Catecholamines are substances that contain catechol (o-dihydroxybenzene) and a side chain with an amino group—the catechol nucleus . Epinephrine is synthesized and stored in the adrenal medulla and released into the systemic circulation. Norepinephrine is synthesized and stored not only in the adrenal medulla but also in the peripheral sympathetic nerves. Dopamine, the precursor of nor epinephrine, is found in the adrenal medulla and peripheral sympathetic nerves.

Secretion of these hormones is controlled by the sympathetic nervous system. The targets of these hormones are the adrenergic receptors in the heart, blood vessels, bronchioles, visceral muscle, skeletal muscle, and in the liver, where they promote glycolysis (breakdown of glycogen).

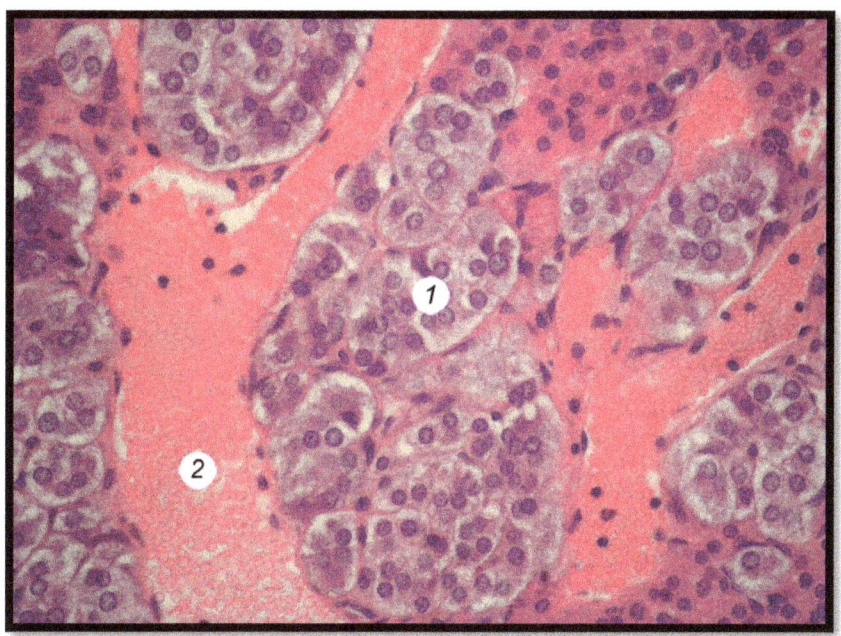

Fig. 18. Rat adrenal gland. Medulla. Control group. Chromaffin cells (1), Expanded medulla veins (2). Hematoxylin and eosin staining, x400

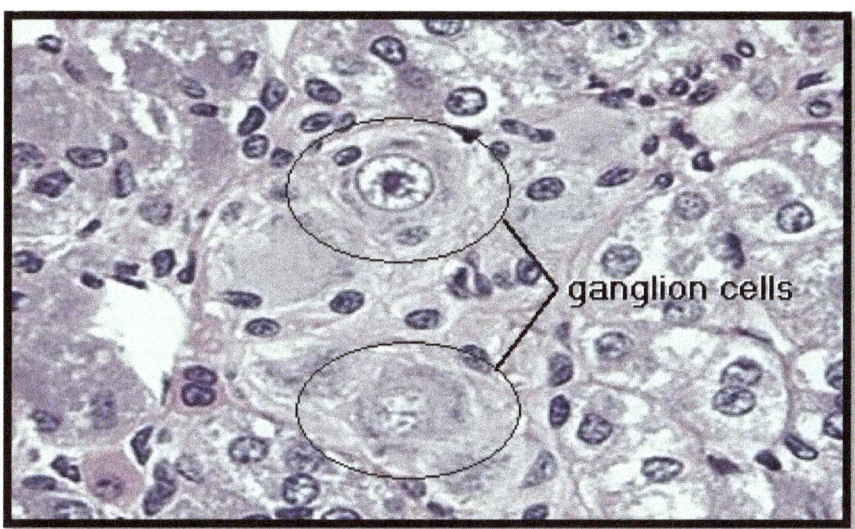

Fig. 19. Enlarged view of the Ganglion cells within the adrenal medulla.

Ultrastructural details of E and NE secreting cells

Adrenomedullary cells in controls had the characteristic ultrastructural features of neuroendocrine cells with an ample presence of membrane bound, secretory ranging from 60 to 400 nm in greatest dimension, and rough endoplasmic reticulum (RER). The catecholamines - epinephrine and nor epinephrine are the major hormones secreted by the adrenal medulla. Norepinephrine is stored in large granules with a dense eccentric core (arrows), whereas epinephrine is stored in smaller granules with a less dense central core (arrowheads). Up to 3 millions molecules of catecholamines are concentrated within a single granule. This large store of catecholamines "floods" the system within seconds after the onset of stress or emergency, exerting on most cells a variety of effects that prepare the body for "fight or flight".

The control chromaffin cells contained large, round nuclei. The cytoplasm contained numerous membrane-bound granules. Cells storing norepinephrine consisted of large-sized granules, with eccentric electron-dense cores. Cells storing epinephrine contained small-sized granules, with concentric less electron-dense cores . Mitochondria, appearing as elongated shapes, well developed rER and Golgi apparatus structures. Nucleus (Nu), an invagination of nuclear membrane (a black arrow), mitochondria (black arrowheads), disrupted cristae of mitochondria (MD), rER (white arrowheads), chromaffin vesicles (CV), degenerated chromaffin vesicles (VD), lysosome (Ly), Golgi apparatus (G), loss of cell organelles (black asterisks). observed .

Ultrastructure of the NE secreting cells of the Adrenal medulla

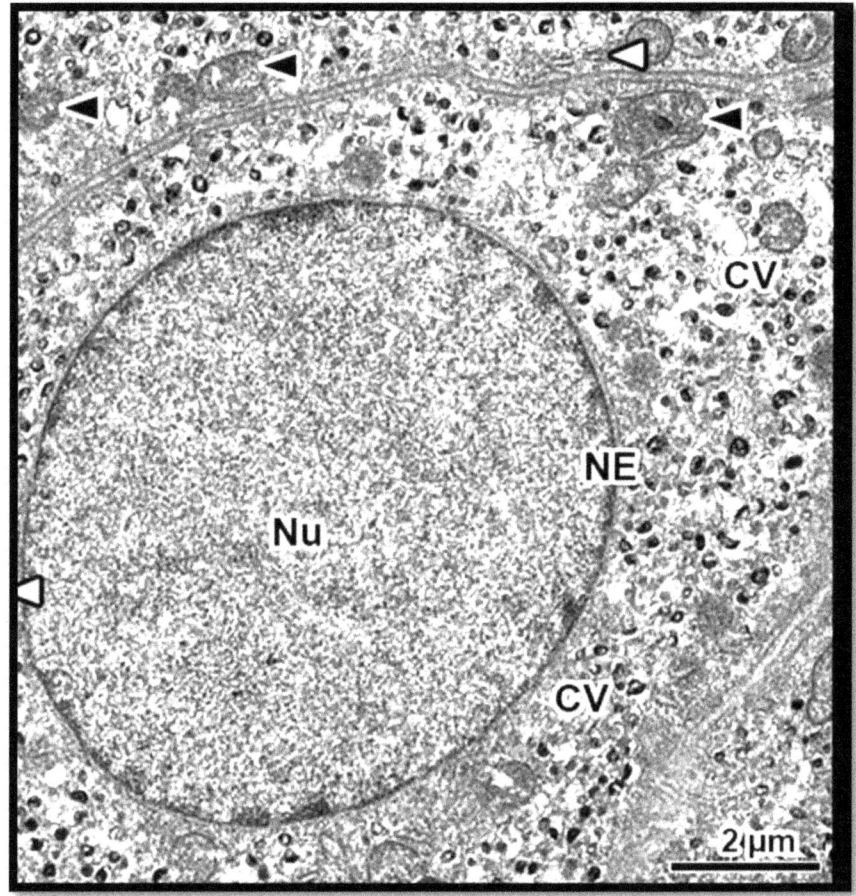

Fig. 20. Ultra structure of Norepinephrine secreting cell of rat ; NE : Nor Epinephrine secreting cell ; NE granules ; CV : chromaffin vesicle ; Nu :Nucleus ; Black arrow head : pointing to the mitochondria ; White arrow head : pointing to rER

Ultrastructure of the E secreting cells of the Adrenal medulla

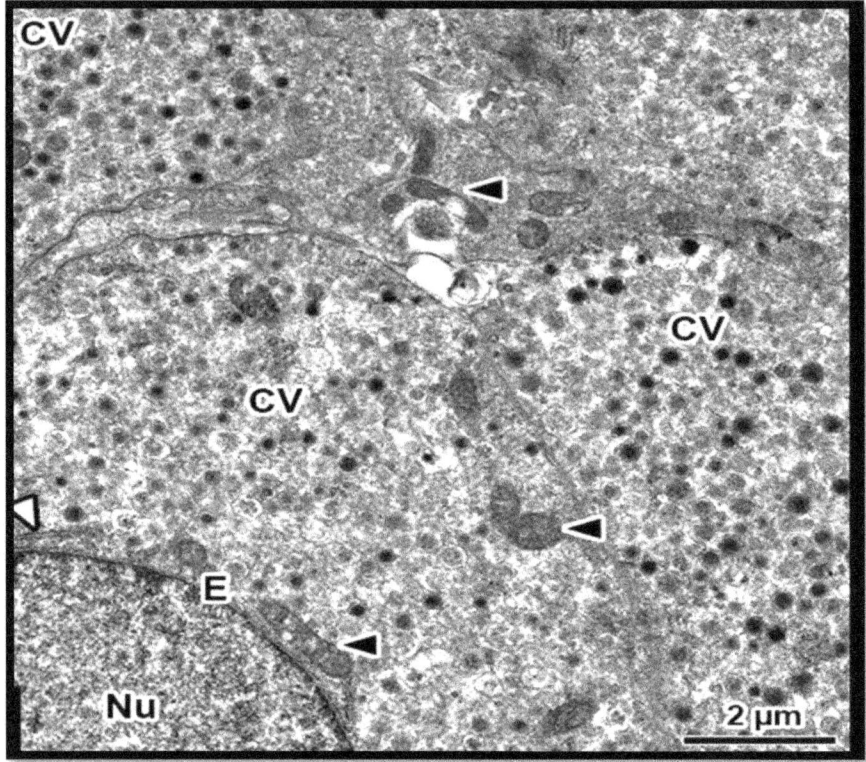

Fig. 21. Structure of Epinephrine (E) secreting cells within the rat adrenal medulla Nu: Nucleus ; E : Epinephrine secreting cell ; CV : Chromaffin vesicle ; Black arrow head : pointing to the mitochondria ; White arrow head : pointing to the rER (rough endoplasmic reticulum).

CONTRIBUTION OF SCIENTISTS ON ADRENAL MEDULLA FUNCTION

A. Sir Edward Albert Sharpey-Schafer

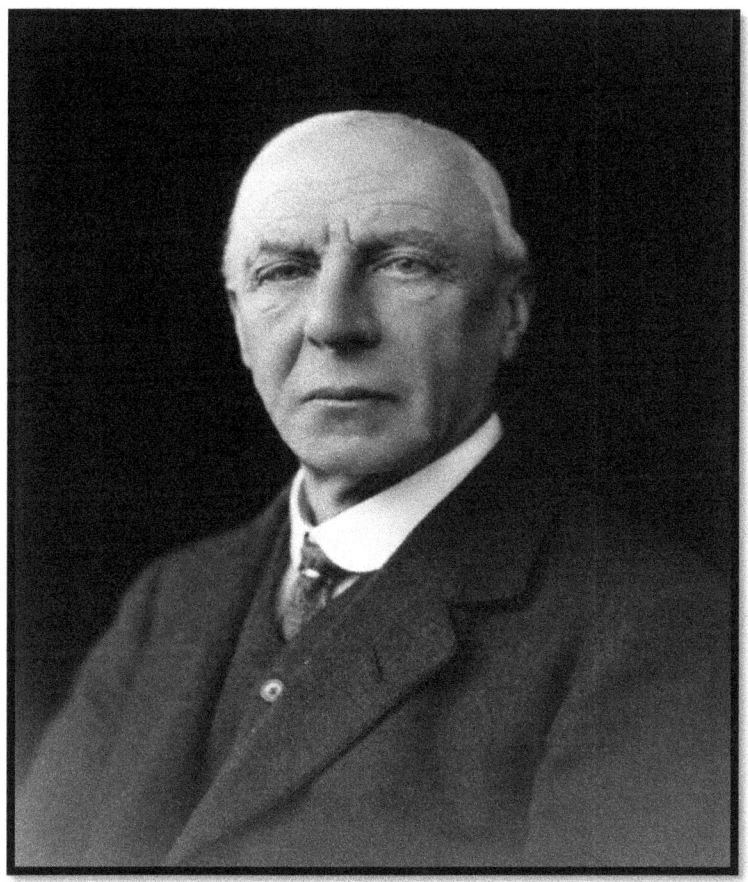

Sir Edward Albert Sharpey-Schafer

Sir Edward Albert Sharpey-Schafer FRS FRSE FRCP LLD was an English physiologist.

Born: 2 June 1850, Hornsey, London, United Kingdom

Died: 29 March 1935, North Berwick, United Kingdom

Known for: Insulin, Endocrine system

English physiologist and inventor of the prone-pressure method (Schafer method) of artificial respiration adopted by the Royal Life Saving Society.

Contribution

He is regarded as a founder of endocrinology: in 1894 he discovered and demonstrated the existence of adrenaline together with George Oliver, and he also coined the term "endocrine" for the secretions of the ductless glands.

Schäer made his most notable contributions in the field of endocrinology, and his papers with George Oliver on the effects of suprarenal of pituitary extracts are landmarks in the history of physiology. The two men showed that while most were inactive, intravenous injections of suprarenal extract produced a dramatic rise in arterial blood pressure, arterial constriction, vagal stimulation (reflex, as we now know), and an increase in the rate and force of cardiac contraction in vagotomized animals. They also pointed out that these effects derived from the medulla, not from the cortex of the gland. They then demonstrated the pressor effect of pituitary extract given intravenously.

B. John Jacob Abel

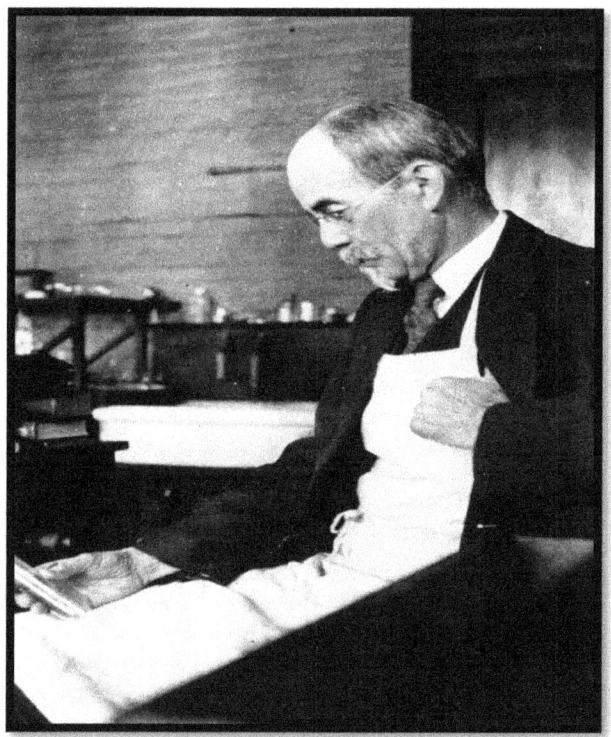

John Jacob Abel

Born : May 19, 1857, Cleveland, Ohio, U.S.

Died : May 26, 1938, Baltimore, Maryland

American pharmacologist and physiological chemist who made important contributions to a modern understanding of the ductless, or endocrine, glands.

Contribution :

Abel's research was mainly biochemical in nature. In 1895 scientists in London had injected an extract from adrenal glands into animals and found that it produced an instant and marked rise in blood pressure. Between 1895 and 1905 Abel worked on isolating the active substance that was found in this gland. In 1897 Abel announced that he had managed to isolate, though not in its pure form, the active substance, which he called epinephrine. He also invented a primitive artificial kidney.

C. Jokichi Takamine

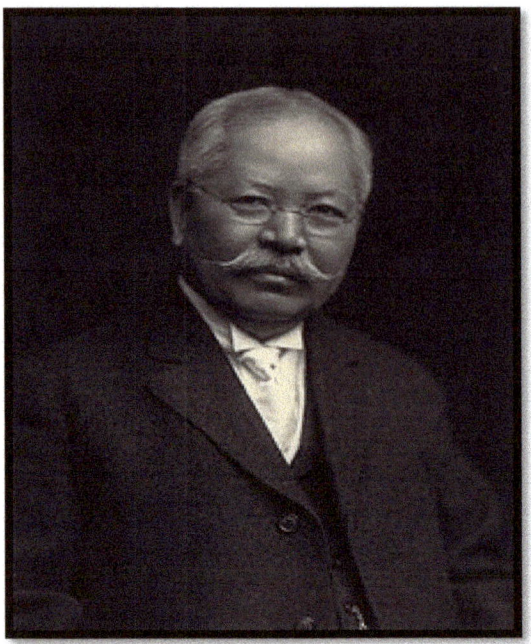

Jokichi Takamine

born : Nov. 3, 1854, Takaoka, Japan

died : July 22, 1922, New York, N.Y., U.S.

Biochemist and industrial leader whose most important achievement was the isolation of the chemical adrenalin (now called epinephrine) from the suprarenal gland (1901). This was the first pure hormone to be isolated from natural sources.

Major contribution

In 1900, Takamine, together with his assistant Keizo Uenaka, was trying to isolate the active principle from the extract of mammalian adrenal glands in a private laboratory in New York, that was affiliated to a pharmaceutical company, Parke Davies. Six years before, G. Oliver and E.A. Schäfer had discovered that the extract of mammalian adrenal glands exerts a powerful hypertensive action on blood pressure. Based on this observation, trials to isolate the active principle were made by J.J. Abel, O. von Fürth and Takamine in a competitive setting.

NOBEL PRIZE

Noradrenaline : Fate and Control of Its Biosynthesis

The Nobel Prize in Physiology or Medicine 1970
1. Sir Bernard Katz
2. Ulf von Euler
3. Julius Axelrod

Sir Bernard Katz

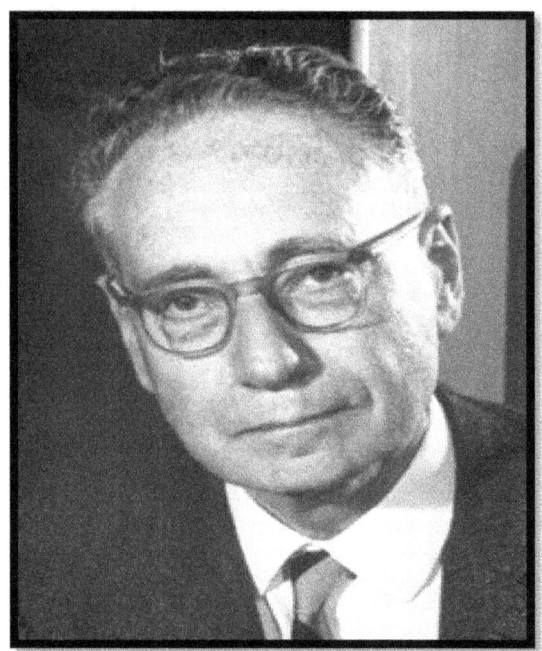

Sir Bernard Katz

The Nobel Prize in Physiology or Medicine 1970

Born : 26 March 1911, Leipzig, Germany

Died : 20 April 2003, London, United Kingdom

Affiliation at the time of the award: University College, London, United Kingdom

Contribution

The major fields of research of Professor Katz include: studies of nerve and muscle, especially of the physico-chemical mechanism of neuromuscular transmission.

Work

The nervous systems of people and animals consist of many nerve cells with long extensions, or nerve fibers. Signals are conveyed between cells by small electrical currents and by special substances known as signal substances. The transfers occur via contacts, or synapses. In the 1950s Bernard Katz studied how impulses in motor neurons activate muscular activity by measuring variations in electrical charges. For example, he showed how the signal substance acetylcholine in synapses is released in certain amounts.

Ulf von Euler

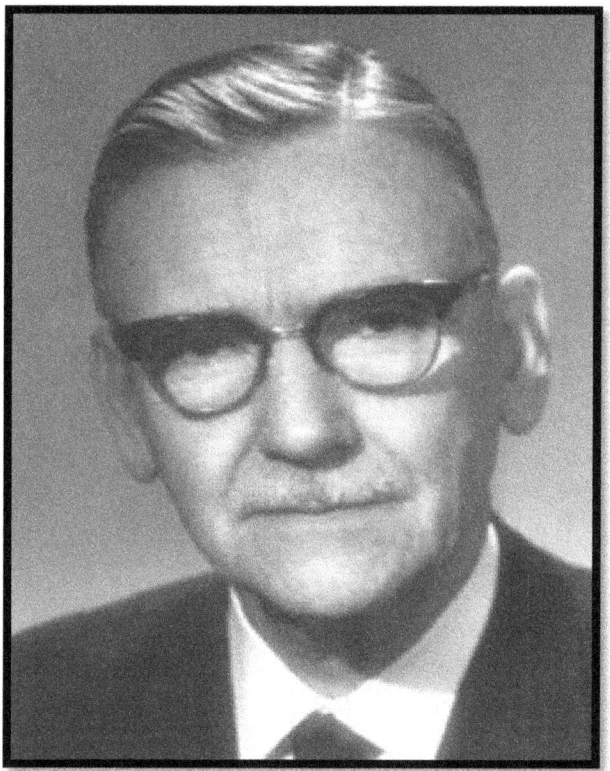

Ulf von Euler

The Nobel Prize in Physiology or Medicine, 1970.
Born: 7 February 1905, Stockholm, Sweden
Died: 9 March 1983, Stockholm, Sweden
Affiliation at the time of the award: Karolinska Institutet, Stockholm, Sweden

Contribution:

Euler's outstanding achievement was his identification of noradrenaline (norepinephrine), the key neurotransmitter (or impulse carrier) in the sympathetic nervous system. He also found that norepinephrine is stored within nerve fibres themselves. These discoveries laid the foundation for Axelrod's determination of the role of the enzyme that inhibits its action, and the method of norepinephrine's reabsorption by nerve tissues. Euler also discovered the hormones known as prostaglandins, which play active roles in stimulating human muscle contraction and in the regulation of the cardiovascular and nervous systems.

Julius Axelrod

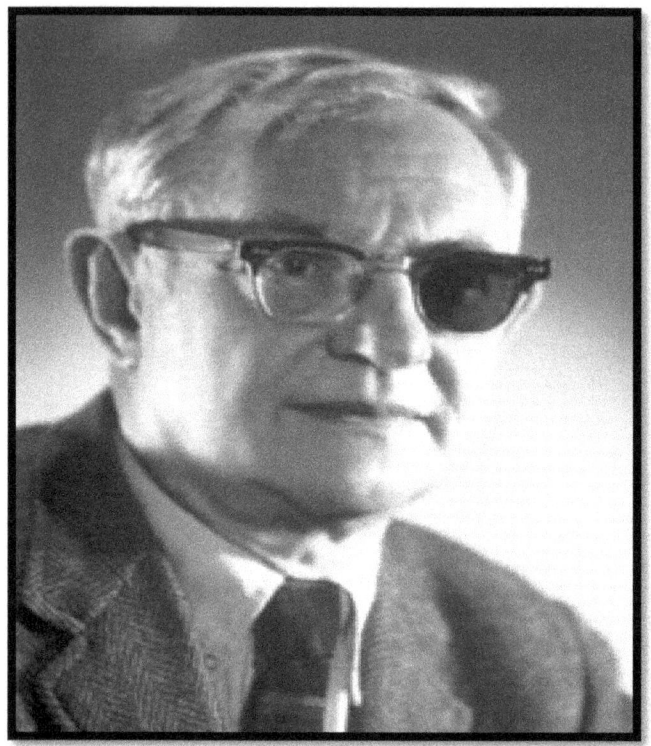

Julius Axelrod

The Nobel Prize in Physiology or Medicine, 1970

Born: 30 May 1912, New York, NY, USA
Died: 29 December 2004, Rockville, MD, USA
Nationality : American
Known for : Catecholamine metabolism

Contribution

Axelrod's Nobel Prize-winning research grew out of work done by Euler, specifically Euler's discovery of noradrenaline (norepinephrine), a chemical substance that transmits nerve impulses. Axelrod, in turn, discovered that noradrenaline could be neutralized by an enzyme, catechol-O-methyltransferase, which he isolated and named. This enzyme proved critical to an understanding of the entire nervous system. The enzyme was shown to be useful in dealing with the effects of certain psychotropic drugs and in research on hypertension and schizophrenia.

TESTIS

ANATOMICAL POSITION OF TESTIS

Male reproductive anatomy

The testes, the male gonads, are large, oval-shaped lobes found in the scrotum slightly anterior to the anus on the ventral side of the organism. Inside the testis are seminiferous tubules where sperm cells are made. When mature, sperm cells travel to and are stored in the epididymis. During ejaculation, sperm are released from the epididymis and travel through the vas deferens to the urogenital duct. Along the sperm's journey through the vas deferens, several glands contribute fluid to the sperm to make semen.

ANATOMICAL POSITION OF TESTIS

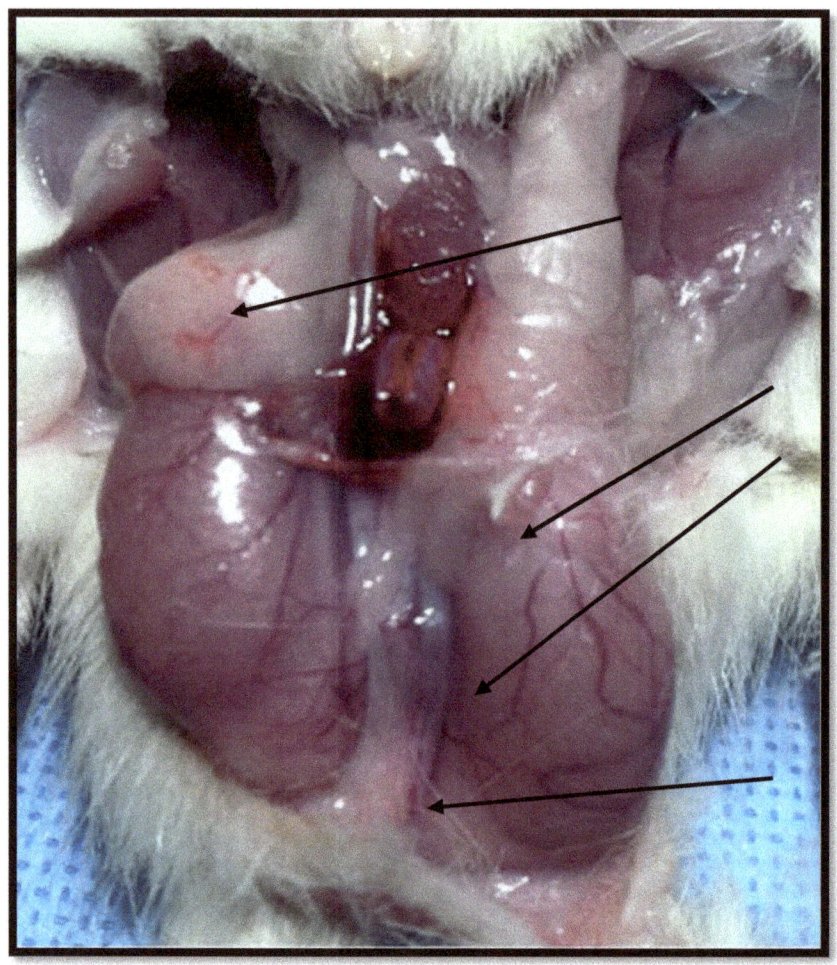

Fig. 22. Representative images exposing rat testes from age-matched 50 day old rats.

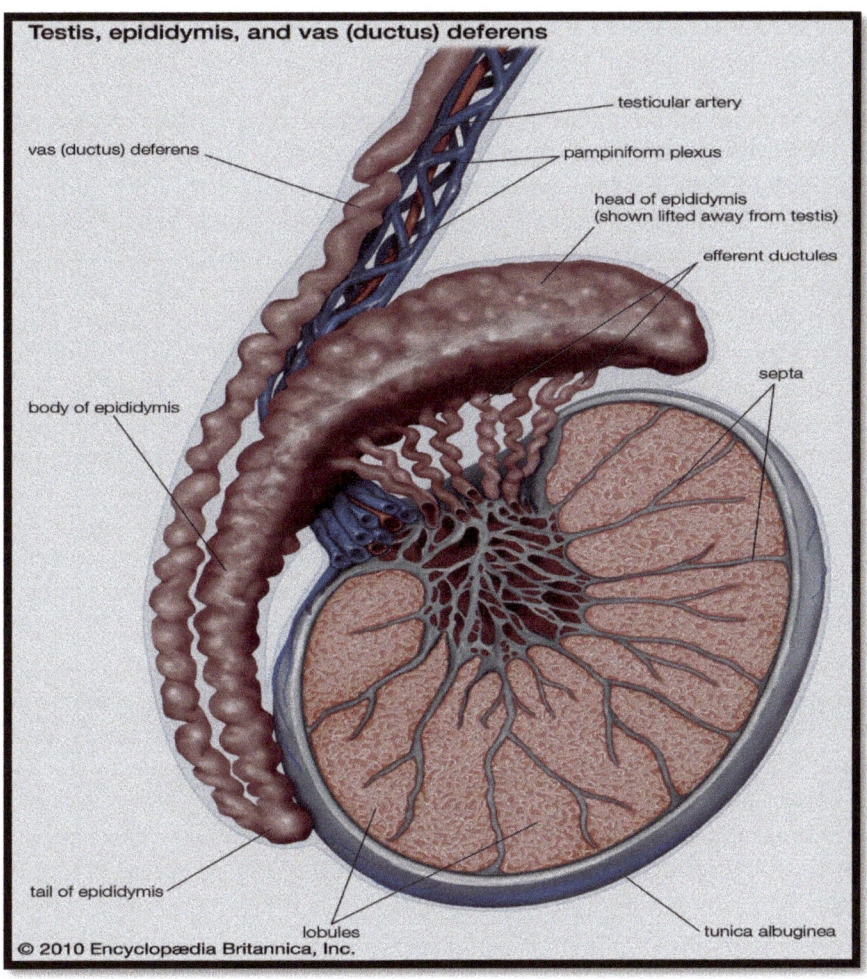

Fig. 23. Diagrammatic presentation of the association of testis, epididymis and vas deferens in rat.

HISTOLOGICAL STRUCTURES OF THE TESTIS

Testes sections of the control rats showed normal histological architecture. The testicular tissue was formed of many tightly packed seminiferous tubules lined by Sertoli cells and germinal epithelium. The germinal epithelium consisted of several layers of spermatogenic cells which are formed of spermatogonia, spermatocytes, spermatids, and sperms. Spermatogonia appeared as small rounded cells with rounded nuclei present in the basal part of the tubules. Primary spermatocytes were larger in size than the spermatogonia with large rounded nuclei. Early spermatids appeared as small rounded cells with paler nuclei. Sperms were demonstrated by their long tails in the lumen of tubules. Sertoli cells appeared pyramidal in shape with large vesicular nuclei and prominent nucleoli. Each tubule was ensheathed by a definite basement membrane and surrounded by flattened myoid cells with flattened nuclei. The narrow interstitial spaces in between the tubules were occupied by the connective tissue and clusters of Leydig cells with acidophilic cytoplasm and vesicular nuclei .

In a cross section of a seminiferous tubule, the germ cells are arranged in discrete layers. Spermatogonia lie on the basal lamina, spermatocytes are arranged above them and then one or two layers of spermatids above them. In any given normal tubule, four generations of cells develop simultaneously and in precise synchrony with each other. As each generation develops, it moves up through the epithelium, continuously supported by Sertoli cells, until the fully formed sperm are released into the tubular lumen (spermiation). The synchrony of the development between the 4 generations of cells is such that each successive stage of development of the spermatogonium is found with its characteristic spermatocyte and spermatids.

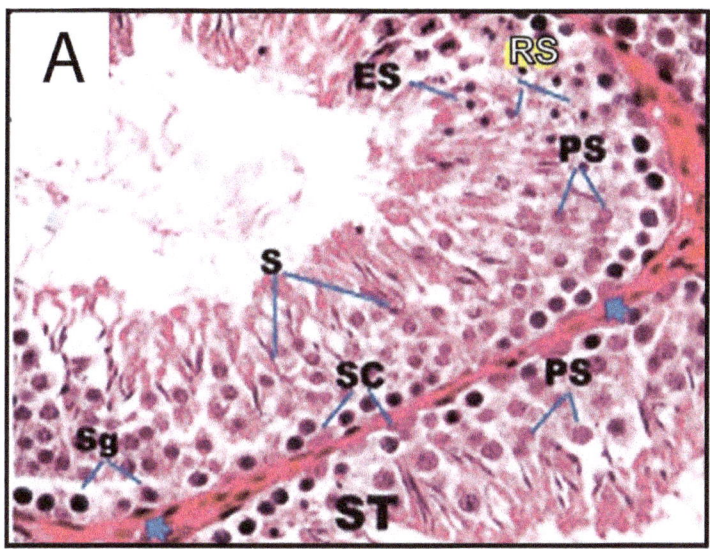

Fig. 24. Histological structure of rat testis as assessed in paraffin sections. Hematoxylin and eosin staining. A. Control rat. Normal shape of seminiferous tubules (ST) with normal arrangement of spermatogonia (Sg) and Sertoli cells (SCs) resting on intact basement membrane (arrowhead). Typical structure of primary spermatocytes (Ps), round (RS) and elongated spermatids (ES) and late stage sperms (S) at the apices of SCs (Johnsen-like score 10); Magnifications: × 400

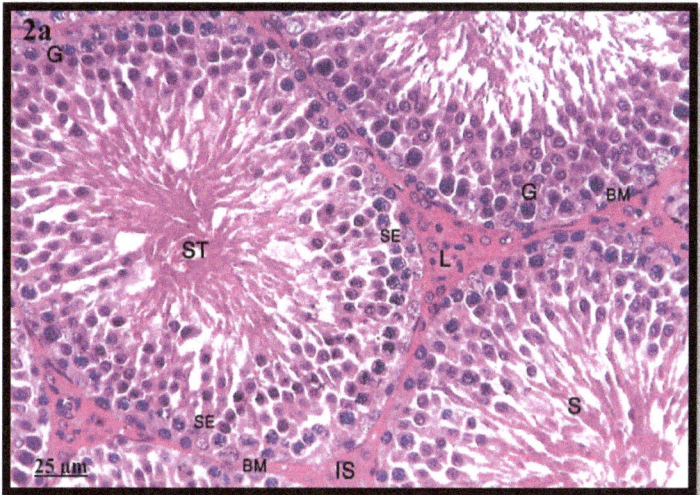

Fig. 25. A photomicrograph of a section in the testis of rat showing normal seminiferous tubules (ST) lined by germinal epithelium (G) and Sertoli cells (SE) resting on the basement membrane (BM). Sperms (S) are seen in the lumen. Notice narrow normal interstitial spaces (IS) in between the tubules, which contain interstitial cells of Leydig (L) (H and E, × 400, scale bar = 25 μm) .

Blood-Testis Barrier (BTB)

The BTB provides a unique microenvironment in the adluminal (apical) compartment of the seminiferous epithelium that is composed of Sertoli and germ cells only, and it is also considered to contribute, at least in part, to the immune-privileged status of the testis by preventing autoantigens residing in late spermatocytes and postmeiotic germ cells from being recognized by the host immune cells. However, this immunological barrier can be leaky in that many germ cell autoantigens also reside in spermatogonia and early spermatocytes that are found outside the BTB. Collectively, these findings show that perhaps the immunosuppressive biomolecules secreted by Sertoli cells are more important in conferring immune privilege status to the testis.

Ultrastructure of the testis

Ultrastructural analysis of the testes of control animals showed that the Sertoli cells and germ cells had cellular characteristics typical of those seen in active spermatogenesis. The Sertoli cells of control animals showed distinct nuclear and cytoplasmic characteristics consistent with an active secretory state. The nuclei were irregular, with patchy chromatin material, deep indentations and well-defined nucleoli. Adjacent to the nuclei, the cytoplasm was characterized by cisternae of rough endoplasmic reticulum, in close association with lipid droplets. Mitochondria were well defined and scattered throughout the cytoplasm. Golgi bodies were also well defined, and free ribosomes and glycogen granules were dispersed throughout the cytoplasm. The plasma membranes were conspicuous and tortuous, showing close associations with adjacent spermatocytes and spermatids. Secretory granules were abundant. The spermatocytes, both primary and secondary, displayed round configurations with prominent nuclei. The nuclei contained distinct chromatin networks in the process of condensation and well-defined nuclear membranes.

The cytoplasm of the primary spermatocytes appeared granular, characterized by dispersed mitochondria and loose networks of rough endoplasmic reticulum.

Cytoplasmic organelles of the secondary spermatocytes were relatively sparse.

Round spermatids were characterized by well-defined nuclei with distinct nuclear membranes and chromatin networks, and their cytoplasm was occupied predominantly with mitochondria. Formation of acrosome aggregations, marked by Golgi vesicles, appeared normal.

The Leydig cells showed distinct nuclear characteristics. The cytoplasm showed prominent lipid bodies, well-defined vesicles of smooth endoplasmic reticulum and mitochondria surrounding the nucleus.

BLOOD TESTIS BARRIER

The blood–testis barrier is a physical barrier between the blood vessels and the seminiferous tubules of the testes. The term is a bit misleading as it is not a blood-organ barrier, but rather one that is formed by the tight junctions between Sertoli cells of the seminiferous tubules. For this reason, this barrier is also referred to as the "Sertoli cell barrier". The barrier isolates further developed germ cells from the blood.

The presence of the blood-testis barrier allows Sertoli cells to control the environment in which germ cells (i.e., spermatocytes, spermatids, and sperm) develop. It also prevents toxins from entering the seminiferous tubules, protecting the germ cells as they develop. The fluid in the open space of the seminiferous tubules (called the lumen) is different from the plasma in blood. It contains very little protein and glucose, and is rather composed of androgens, estrogens, and other substances. The blood-testis barrier helps maintain this unique chemical composition.

Functions of blood-testis barrier:
1. Selects the nutrients, hormones and other structures needed for the spermatogenic cells.
2. Isolates and protects the spematogenic cells from any damaging materials, antigen or antibodies in the circulating blood.
3. Prevents leakage of testicular fluid and androgen- binding protein secreted by Sertoli cells to the interstitial tissues.

ULTRASTRUCTURE

The Sertoli Cells and Their Junctional Complexes.

The germinal epithelium of the testis is composed of a fixed population of supporting Sertoli cells, a stem cell population of spermatogonia resting on the basal lamina, and a mobile population of developing germ cells whose topographical relations to the fixed elements are constantly changing as these cells differentiate and are displaced upward toward the lumen. As might be expected, specializations for attachment do not develop on the surfaces of contact between germ cells and supporting cells, for presumably these would interfere with the upward mobility of the germ cells. There are, however, enduring contacts and specialized junctions between adjacent members of the fixed population of supporting cells.

Indeed, the formation of these junctional specializations and their extension may be a means by which the clones of germ cells are moved upward in the epithelium.

A double membrane, cup-shaped structure known as the phagophore appeared within the cytoplasm of the SCs. This cup-shaped structure invigilates the cytoplasm of SCs, inside the double membrane . Electron microscopic imaging revealed a unique structure known as the cytoplasmic bridge between the two spermatids, which was composed of SCs. The SCs surrounded the head of the spermatid during the development of the acrosomal cap and contained an abundance of endoplasmic reticulum. This endoplasmic reticulum exhibited many tubules and dense material secreted at the site of the acrosomal cap .

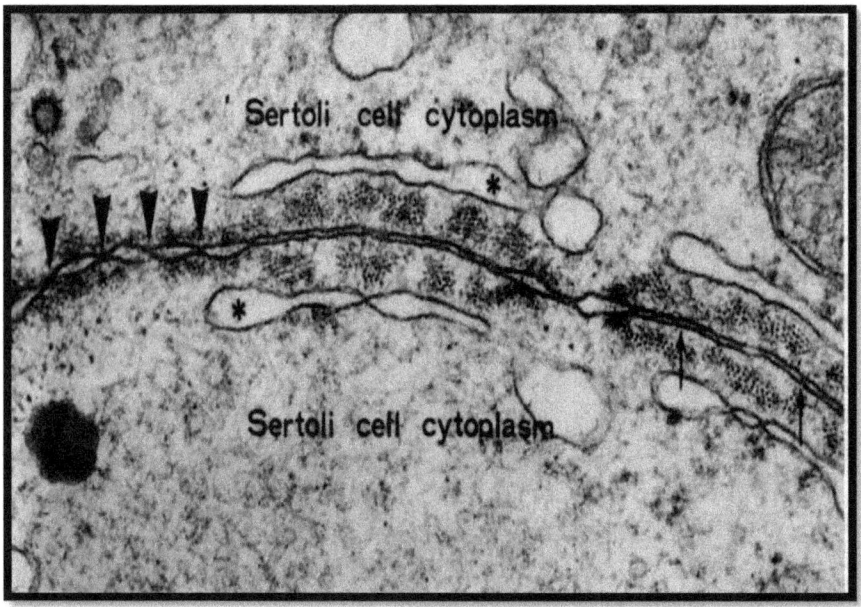

Fig. 26. Electron micrograph of a Sertoli-Sertoli intercellular junction. Tight junctions (arrowheads) and 90-A "narrow" junctions (arrows) are apparent. Subsurface cisternae of endoplasmic reticulum (*) are separated from the cell surface by bundles of filaments that are hexagonally arranged. X63,000.

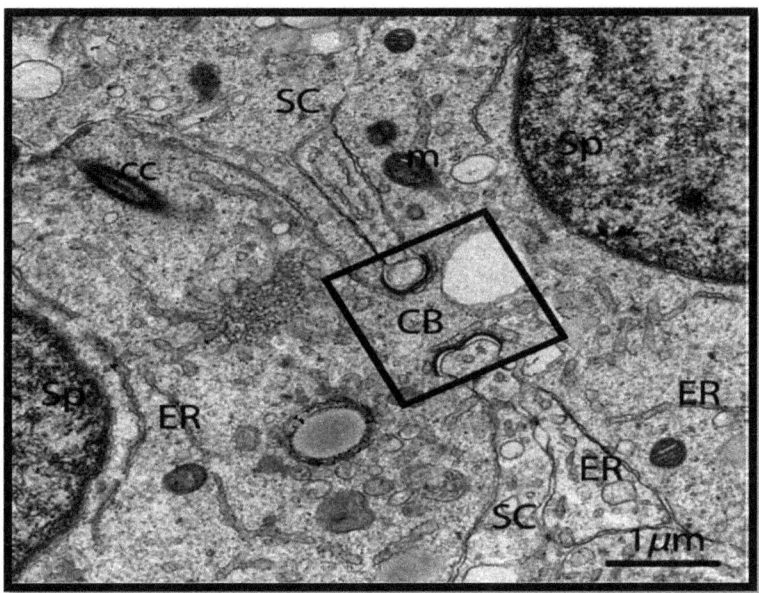

Fig. 27. Electron micrograph of a Sertoli cell that exhibits the cytoplasmic bridge (rectangular area) . SC, Sertoli cell; Sp, spermatid; CB, cytoplasmic bridge; ER, endoplasmic reticulum; m: mitochondria; CC, centrosome. Scale bar = 1 μm.

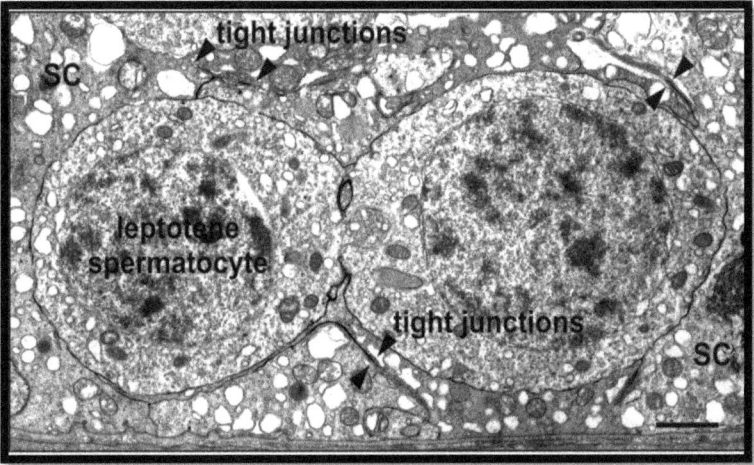

Fig. 28. An electron micrograph of the intermediate compartment in the adult rat testis. This image shows 2 leptotene spermatocytes connected by intercellular bridges and enclosed within the intermediate compartment at stages IX–XI of the seminiferous epithelial cycle. The blood testis barrier, which is created by Sertoli cells (SCs), is visible by the precipitation of lanthanum nitrate (arrowheads), which fails to advance beyond the TJs. Scale bar, 1 μm. (Reproduced from Mruk and Cheng and used with permission.)

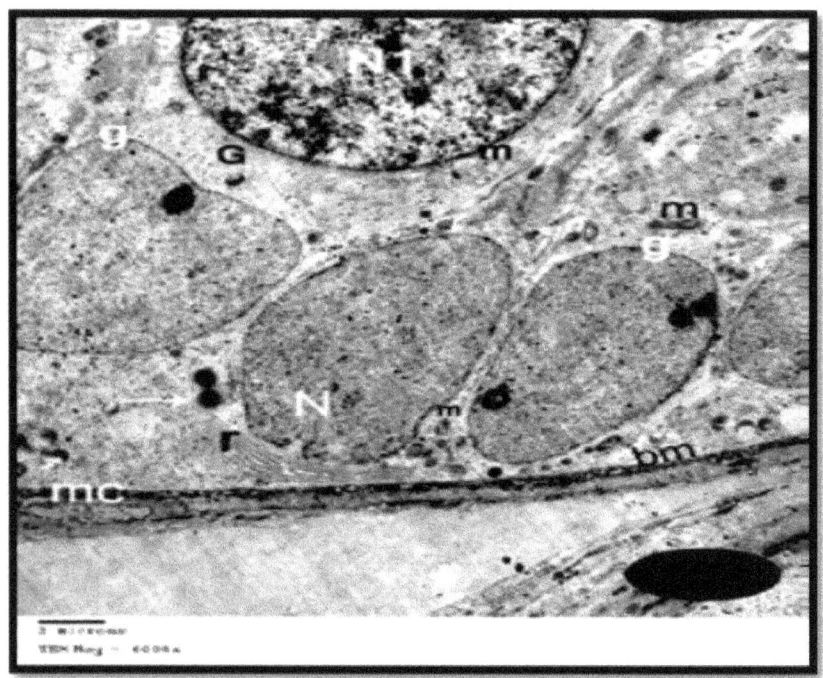

Fig. 29. An electron micrograph of testis of control group I showing a part of a seminiferous tubule surrounded by a regular basement membrane (bm) and ensheathed by a myoid cell (mc). Spermatogonia (g) appear with rounded, oval euchromatic nuclei and mitochondria (m). Primary spermatocyte (Ps) with part of a large rounded nucleus containing clumps of heterochromatin (N1) can be observed. Its cytoplasm contains mitochondria (m) and free small ribosomal granules (G). Sertoli cell with indented a euchromatic nucleus (N) and its cytoplasm containing cisternae of endoplasmic reticulum (r), mitochondria (m) and electrondense bodies (arrow) in the basal part of its cytoplasm can be observed. × 6000.

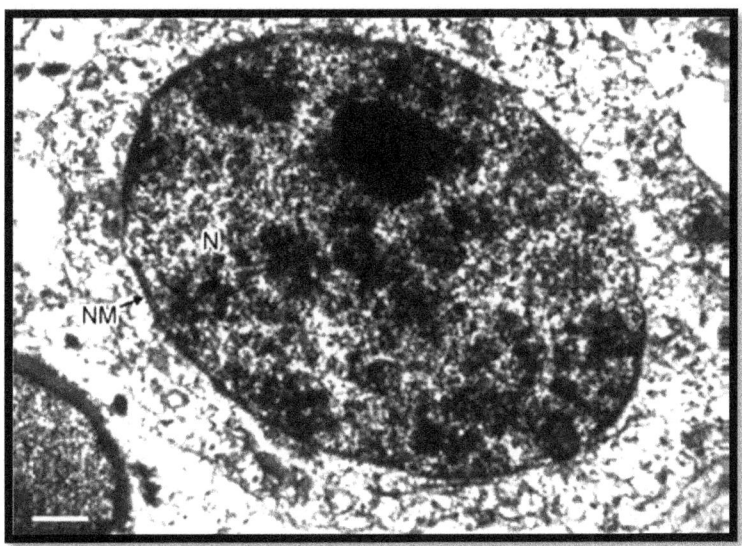

Fig. 30. Ultrastructure of the testis of control animals showing the primary spermatocytes. The cytoplasm appears granular. The nucleus contains distinct chromatin networks, with well-defined nucleoli and prominent nuclear membranes. Scale bar = 2.17 µm. N, nucleus ; NM, nuclear membrane.

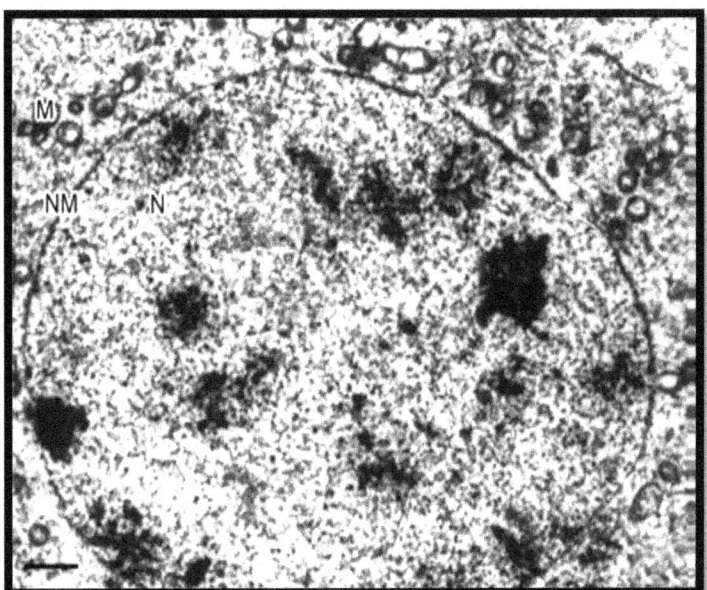

Fig. 31. Ultra structure of the testis of control animals, showing a secondary spermatocyte. The nucleus contains condensed chromatin material and a distinct nuclear membrane. Mitochondria are scattered throughout the cytoplasm. M, mitochondria; N, nucleus; NM, nuclear membrane. Scale bar = 2.17 µm.

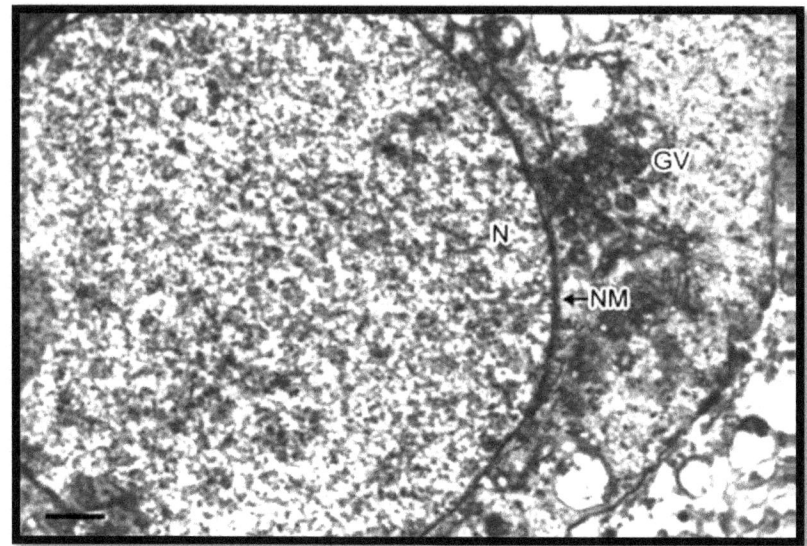

Fig. 32. Ultrastructure of the testis of control animals showing a round spermatid. The nucleus is round, with a prominent nuclear membrane. Mitochondria occupy the periphery of the cytoplasm. Golgi vesicles are well defined. GV, Golgi vesicles; N, nucleus; NM, nuclear membrane. Scale bar = 2.78 μm.

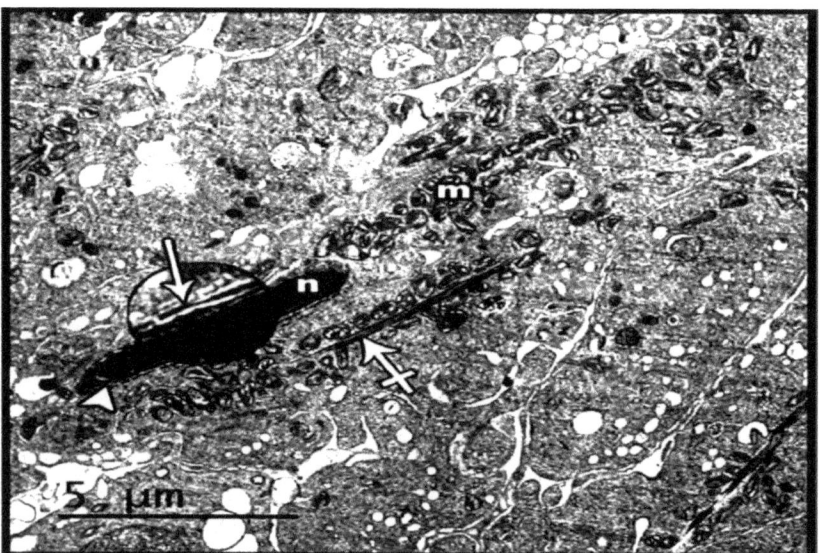

Fig. 33. An electron micrograph of control rat testis showing two sperms, the upper one has elongated condensed nucleus (*n*) and acrosomal cap (arrow head) at the leading point of the head. The middle piece of the flagellum contains numerous mitochondria (*m*). Note ectoplasmic specialization (arrow). The lower one shows the axoneme (crossed arrow) surrounded with mitochondrial sheath (TEM, ×10,000).

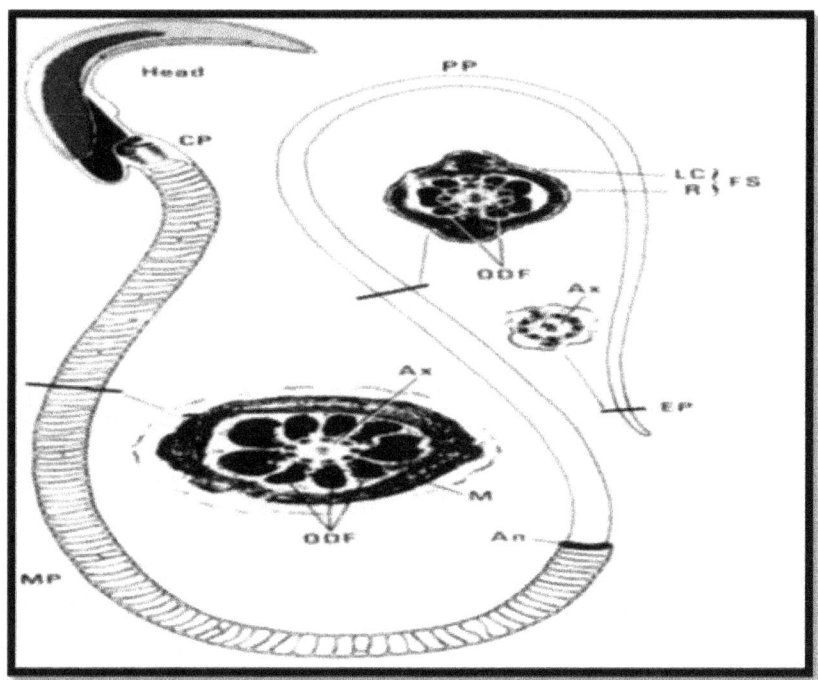

Fig. 34. Schematic representation of a rat spermatozoon (left) with a sickle shaped head and long tail. The tail consists of the connecting piece (CP), middle (MP), principal (PP) and end (EP) pieces and annulus (An) at the junction of the middle and principal piece. Cross section of the middle piece reveals the central axoneme (Ax), and nine outer dense fibers (ODF) and peripherally located mitochondrial sheath (M). Cross section of the principal piece reveals the presence of the fibrous sheath (FS) consisting of the longitudinal columns (LC) and transverse ribs (R).

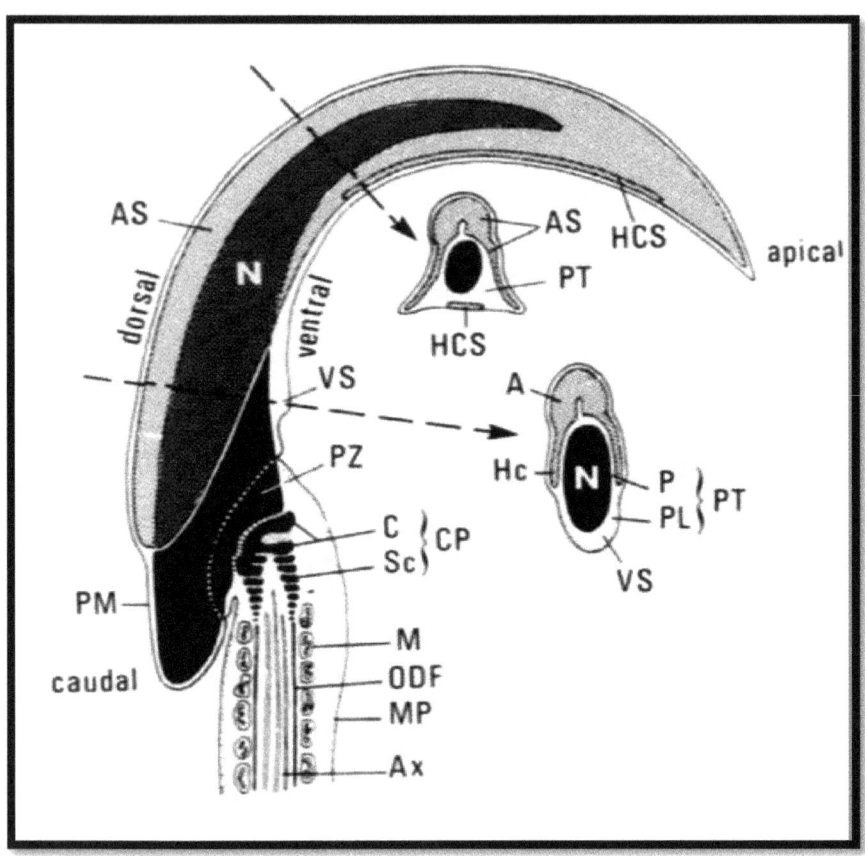

Fig. 35. Labeled in the rat sperm head are: PM, plasma membrane; N, nucleus; AS, acrosomic system (A , acrosome ; Hc , head cap ; HCS , separated head cap segment , ES , equatorial segment) ; PT , perinuclear theca (P, perforatorium ; PL , postacrosomal lamina) ; PZ , perifossal zone and CP connecting piece (C, capitulum ; Sc , striated columns) . VS , ventral spur. (Reproduced with permission from Clermont et al., Cell and molecular biology of the testis, 1993, pp. 332–376 , Oxford University Press).

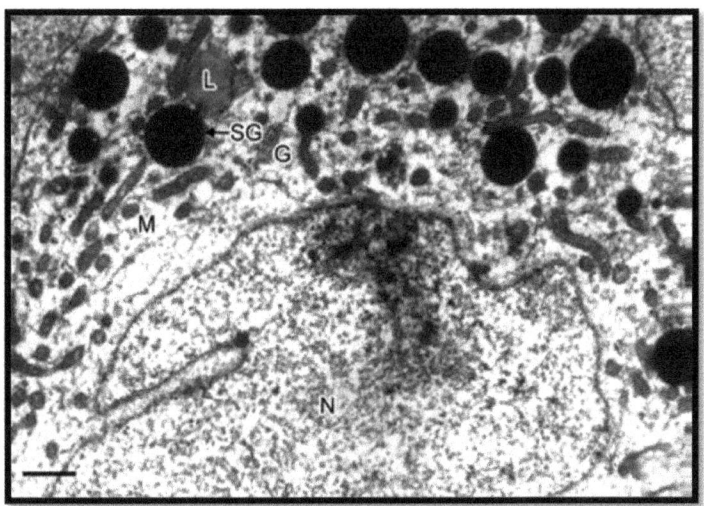

Fig. 36. Ultrastructure of the testis of control animals showing the Sertoli cells. The nucleus appears irregular, with indentations. The cytoplasmic organelles indicate an active secretory state. The mitochondria, lipid droplets and rough endoplasmic reticulum are prominent and scattered throughout the cytoplasm. Secretory granules are abundant. Scale bar = 1.79 µm. G, Golgi bodies; L, lipid droplets; M, mitochondria; N, nucleus; SG, secretory granules.

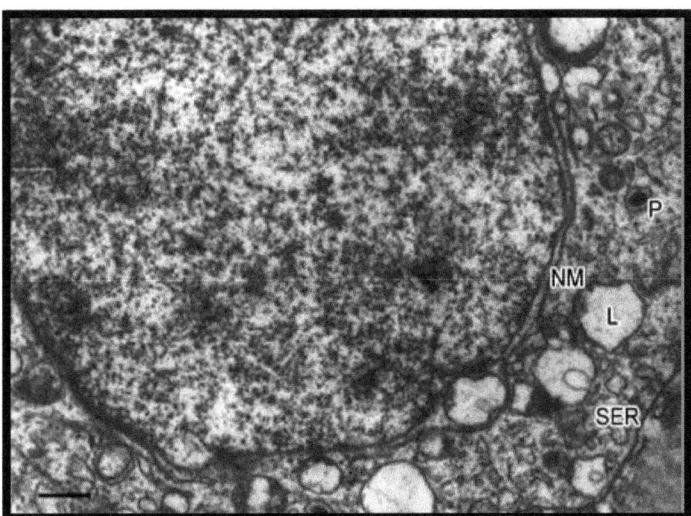

Fig. 37. Ultrastructure of the testis of a control animal, showing a Leydig cell. The cell is characterized by a round nucleus, containing a prominent nuclear membrane. The cytoplasm shows vesicles of smooth endoplasmic reticulum, prosecretory granules, prominent mitochondria and lipid bodies. L, lipid bodies ; NM, nuclear membrane ; P, prosecretory granules ; SER, smooth endoplasmic reticulum. Scale bar = 2.78 µm.

CONTRIBUTION OF SCIENTISTS ON TESTICULAR FUNCTIONS

Professor Enrico Sertoli

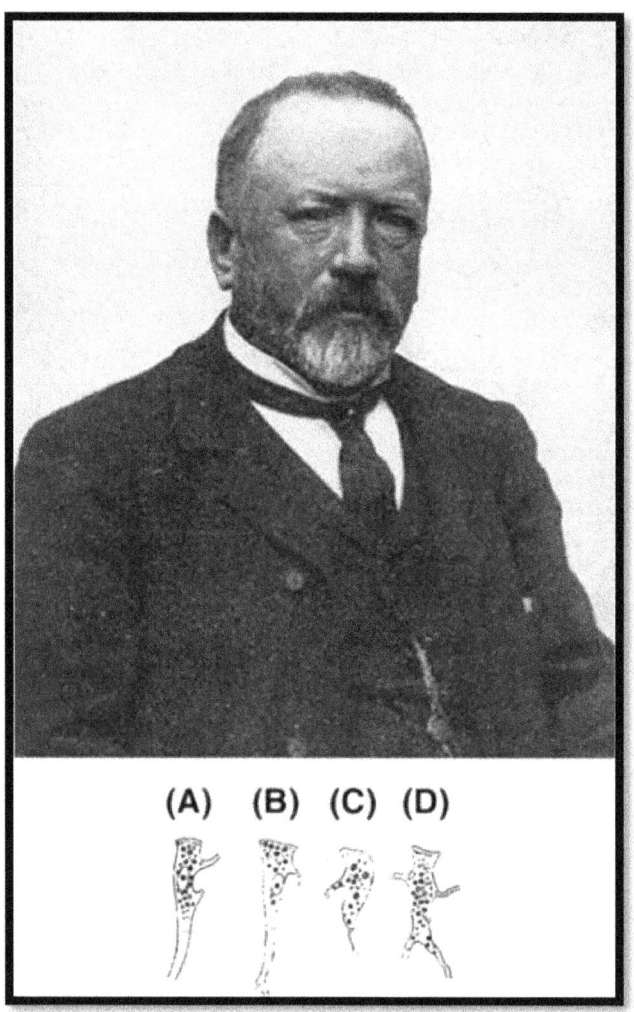

Professor Enrico Sertoli

Born: 6 June 1842, Sondrio, Italy
Died: 28 January 1910, Sondrio, Italy, (aged 67)
Education: The University of Pavia

Contribution of Scientists

Sertoli is remembered for his 1865 discovery of the eponymous Sertoli cell. These cells line the tubuli seminiferi contorti of the testis, and provide nourishment and support for developing sperm.

Ref : Sertoli E. Dell'esistenza di particolari cellule ramificate nei canalicoli seminiferi del testicolo umano. Morgagni. 1865; 7:31–40.

The cellular associations in the mammalian testis have been a subject of discussion since the production of quality microscopes was coupled with inquiring minds. The possiblity of a functional relationship between the 'branched cells' and the production of spermatozoa was first described by Enrico Sertoli when he was a new university graduate at the age of 23.

Sertoli cells play a key role in the regulation of spermatogenesis and the production of spermatozoa.

Franz von Leydig

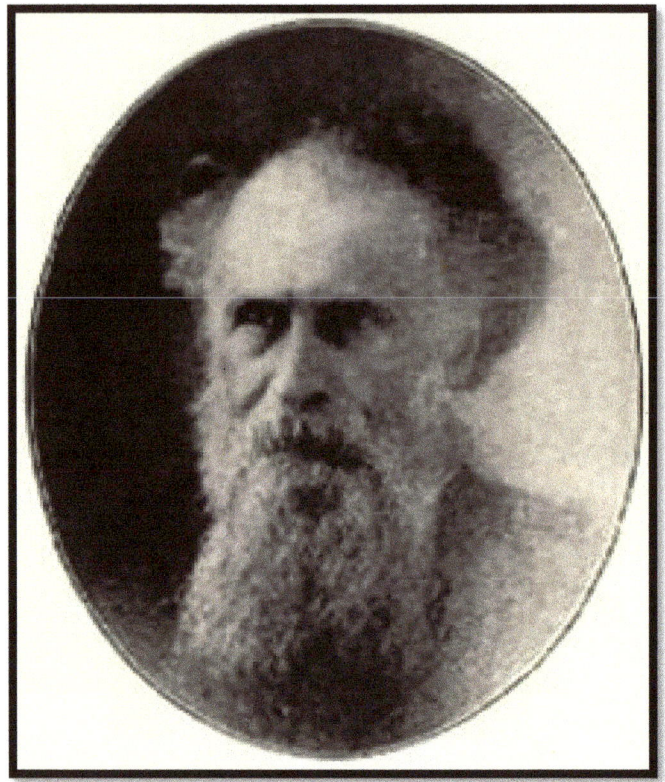

Franz von Leydig

German zoologist and comparative anatomist.

Born : on May 21, 1821

Died : on April 13, 1908, Rothenburg ob der Tauber, Germany (aged 87)

Franz von Leydig, also Franz Leydig ([ˈlaɪdɪç]; May 21, 1821 – April 13, 1908), was a German zoologist and comparative anatomist.

In hormone: Luteinizing hormone (interstitial-cell-stimulating hormone)

…of the interstitial tissue (**Leydig cells**) of the testes and hence promotes secretion of the male sex hormone, testosterone. It may be associated with FSH in this function. The interrelationship of LH and FSH has made it difficult to establish with certainty that two separate hormones exist, particularly since…

The testes contain germ cells that differentiate into mature spermatozoa, supporting cells called Sertoli cells, and testosterone-producing cells called Leydig (interstitial) cells. The germ cells migrate to the fetal testes from the embryonic yolk sac. The Sertoli cells, which are interspersed between the germinal epithelial cells within the seminiferous tubules, are analogous to the granulosa cells in the ovary, and the Leydig cells, which are located beneath the tunica albuginea, in the septal walls, and between the tubules, are analogous to the hormone-secreting interstitial cells of the ovary. The Leydig cells are irregularly shaped and commonly have more than one nucleus. Frequently they contain fat droplets, pigment granules, and crystalline structures; the Leydig cells vary greatly in number and appearance among the various animal species. They are surrounded by numerous blood and lymphatic vessels, as well as by nerve fibres.

Contribution of Scientists

Importance of Leydig cells

Studies of Leydig cells began with the German zoologist and anatomist Franz von Leydig who, in 1850, described the presence of interstitial cells in the testes of several mammals [1, 2]. Fifty years later, Bouin and Ancel first suggested that androgens are produced by the interstitial Leydig cells [3]. About 60 years after that, Baillie demonstrated that these cells contain the enzyme 3β-hydroxysteroid dehydrogenase [4]. At about the same time, Hall and Eik-Nes [5] and Ewing and Eik-Nes [6] showed that pituitary gonadotropic hormones stimulate androgen formation by testes in vitro and ex vivo. In 1969, Hall and colleagues demonstrated that the conversion of cholesterol to testosterone occurred in the interstitial Leydig cells [7]. Thus, from the time of the discovery of interstitial cells in 1850, it took over a century to appreciate the major steps involved in Leydig cell function.

References

1. **Leydig F**. Zur Anatomie der männlichen Geschlechtsorgane und Analdrüsen der Säugethiere. *Zeitschrift f Wiss Zool* 1850;2:1–57.

2. **Le Minor JM, Sick H**. About the 350th anniversary of the foundation of the chair of anatomy of the faculty of medicine at Strasbourg (1652-2002). *Hist Sci Med* 2003;37:31–40.

3. **Bouin P, Ancel P.** Recherches sur les cellules interstitielles du testicle des mammifères. *Arch Zool Exp Gen* 1903;1:437–523.

4. **Baille AH.** Further observations on the growth and histochemistry of Leydig tissue in the postnatal prepubertal mouse testis. *J Anat* 1964;98:403–418.

5. **Hall PF, Eik-Nes KB.** The action of gonadotropic hormones upon rabbit testis in vitro. *Biochim Biophys Acta* 1962;63(3):411–422.

6. **Ewing LL, Eik-Nes KB.** On the formation of testosterone by the perfused rabbit testis. *Can J Biochem* 1966;44(10):1327–1344.

7. **Hall PF, Irby DC, De Kretser DM.** Conversion of cholesterol to androgens by rat testes: comparison of interstitial cells and seminiferous tubules. *Endocrinology* 1969;84(3):488–496.

Butenandt, Adolf

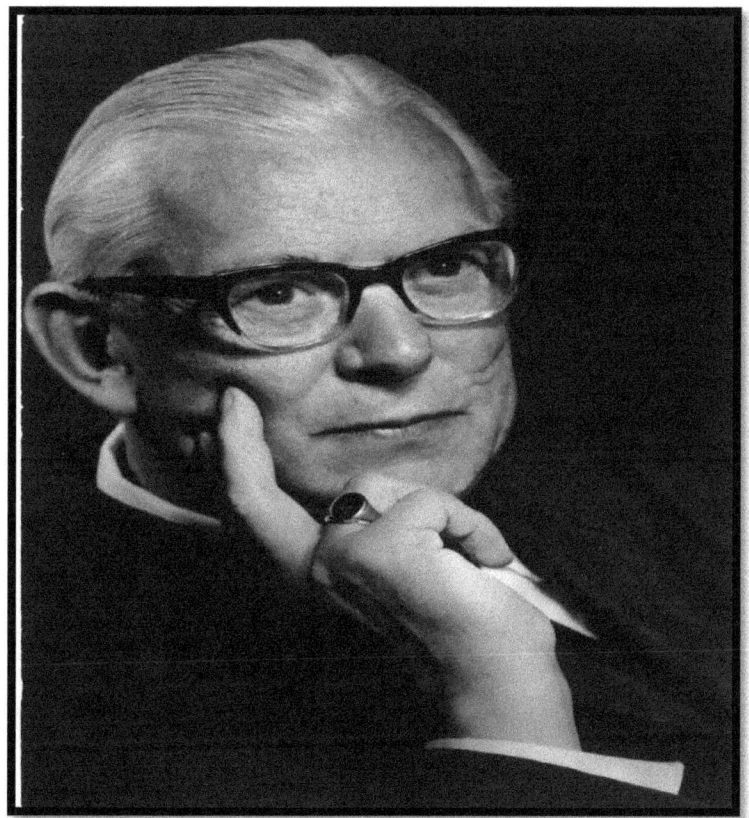

Butenandt, Adolf

Born: March 24, 1903 Germany
Died: January 18, 1995 (aged 91) Munich Germany
Awards And Honors: Nobel Prize (1939)
Subjects Of Study: sex hormone

Contribution

Adolf Butenandt, in full Adolf Friedrich Johann Butenandt, (born March 24, 1903, Bremerhaven-Lehe, Germany—died January 18, 1995, Munich), German biochemist who, with Leopold Ruzicka, was awarded the 1939 Nobel Prize for Chemistry for his work on sex hormones. Although forced by the Nazi government to refuse the prize, he was able to accept the honour in 1949.

In 1929, almost simultaneously with Edward A. Doisy in the United States, Butenandt isolated estrone, one of the hormones responsible for sexual development and function in females. In 1931 he isolated and identified androsterone, a male sex hormone, and in 1934, the hormone progesterone, which plays an important part in the female reproductive cycle. It was now clear that sex hormones are closely related to steroids, and after Ruzicka showed that cholesterol could be transformed into androsterone, he and Butenandt were able to synthesize both progesterone and the male hormone testosterone. Butenandt's investigations made possible the eventual synthesis of cortisone and other steroids and led to the development of birth control pills.

OVARY

ANATOMICAL POSITION OF THE OVARY

Gross Anatomy

The ovaries are the female pelvic reproductive organs that house the ova and are also responsible for the production of sex hormones. They are paired organs located on either side of the uterus within the broad ligament below the uterine (fallopian) tubes. The ovary is within the ovarian fossa, a space that is bound by the external iliac vessels, obliterated umbilical artery, and the ureter. The ovaries are responsible for housing and releasing ova, or eggs, necessary for reproduction.

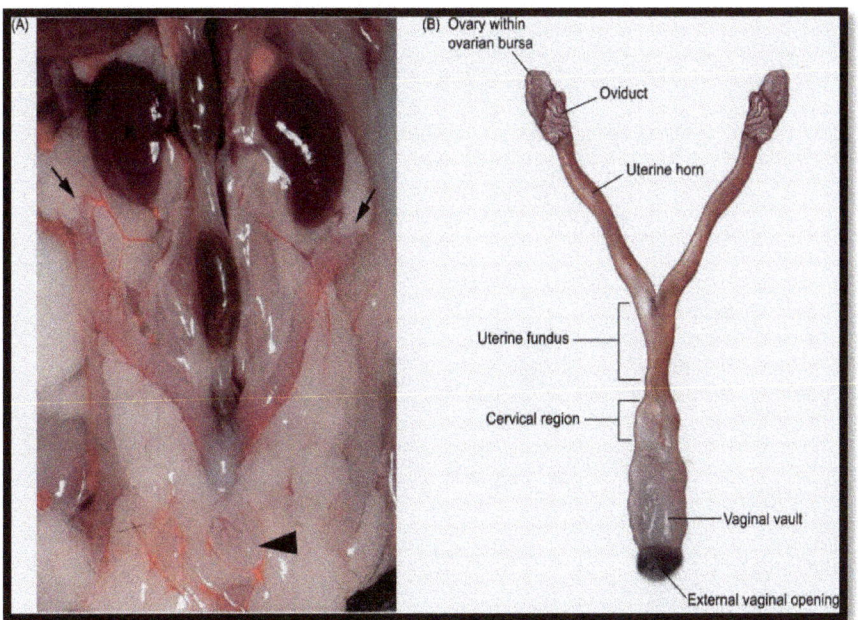

Fig. 38. Anatomical position of the ovary (image from intact rat)

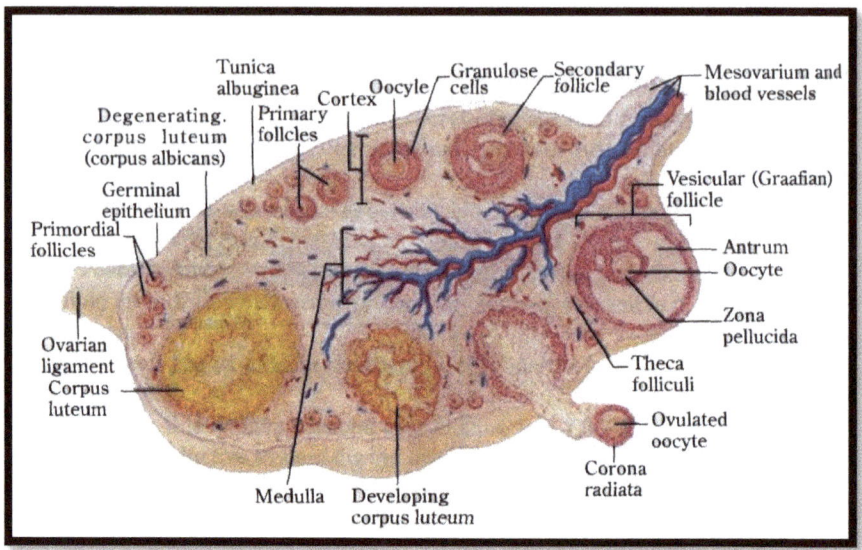

Fig. 39. Transverse section of ovary (Diagrammatic presentation)

HISTOLOGICAL STRUCTURES OF OVARY

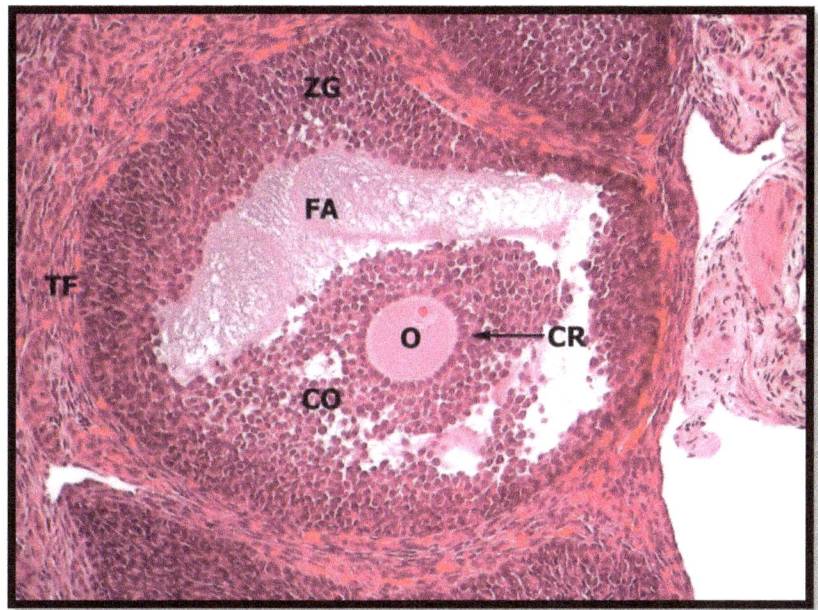

Fig. 40. **Tertiary follicle (rat, H&E x20)**. The large follicular antrum (**FA**) and eccentrically positioned primary oocyte (**O**) characterise this stage. **O** primary oocyte ; **CO** cumulus oophorus ; **CR** corona radiata ; **FA** follicular antrum ; **ZG** zona granulosa ; **TF** theca folliculi

Histopathology of Rat ovarian tissue

Histopathological examination showed that normal histological features in the ovary of the control animal . In control, the ovary was surrounded by germinal epithelium and underline tunica albuginea. Primordial follicles, consist of an oocyte is surrounded by a single layer of squamous follicular cells, primary follicles that consists of an oocyte surrounded by a layer or layers of cuboidal follicular cells were observed. When the follicular cells proliferate into a stratified epithelium known as granulosa cell layer. Secondary follicles with the appearance of a follicular antrum within the granulosa layer were observed.

Different histologic sections of the ovaries from the female control group indicate well development of ovarian follicles, normal blood vessels and normal stroma cells. The pre-ovulatory follicle showed typical morphology of oocyte and euchromatin nucleus, which was surrounded by typical zona pellucida and several layers of granulosa cells are resting on the basement membrane. Theca interna and theca externa are clearly developed. The primary follicles with the normal oocyte surrounded by single layer of cubical granulosa cells are showed to rest on the basement membrane. Hypertrophy of corpus luteum and proliferation and differentiation of steroidogenic cells with extensive angiogenesis are evident .

Ultrastructure of ovarian tissue

Under the electron microscope, the rat ovaries in the control group demonstrated oval-shaped granular cells and basically normal nuclear morphology, with no expansion into the perinuclear space and continuous structure of the **double nuclear membranes**. In addition, there were basically **normal mitochondria** within the cytoplasm, evenly distributed **chromatin** in the nuclei, **long oval mitochondria** in the cytoplasm, **many cristae** in the mitochondria, a moderate amount of **smooth endoplasmic reticulum** and **lipid droplets** in the vacuoles, and a small amount of **rough endoplasmic reticulum** and **Golgi** .

Oocytes in Primordial Follicles

Primordial follicles are composed of an oocyte surrounded by a small number of squamous granulosa cells . Oocytes contained in healthy primordial follicles display lightly staining mitochondria with shelflike cristae, well developed Golgi complexes, and are tightly apposed to the surrounding granulosa cells The nucleus contains small amounts of darkly staining heterochromatin , and large, intact nucleoli with well-developed nucleolonemata are present (not shown).

Oocytes in Healthy Developing Follicles

Ultrastructural morphology of healthy oocytes in developing follicles appears similar regardless of the stage of development. Oocytes in follicles have acquired a zona pellucida. Microvilli from the oocyte and thicker prolongations from granulosa cells penetrate the zona pellucida. The oocyte cytoplasm is sparsely populated with loosely clustered organelles. Mitochondria in oocytes appear round or oval, rather dark, and have small numbers of identifiable shelflike cristae. Very small amounts of rough endoplasmic reticulum (RER) are located adjacent to clusters of mitochondria and are uniformly filled with faintly electrondense material . Vacuoles or lysosomes are rarely observed in oocytes of healthy follicles. The nucleus of developing follicles was never observed to display condensed chromatin outside of the nucleolus and had little electron-dense material .

Light Microscopic Luteal Changes in the rat ovary

During the diestrus stage, the control group produced luteal cells of the new CL, which exhibited pale eosinophilic staining in the cytoplasm with sparse and fine vacuolation ; while the luteal cells of the old CL exhibited strong eosinophilic staining in the cytoplasm and the additional presence of interstitial cells, such as endothelial cells and fibroblasts .

Formation of Corpus luteum

Following extrusion of the secondary oocyte from the Graafian follicle, the granulosa and thecal cells of the follicle remnant undergo hypertrophy and, to a lesser extent, hyperplasia. This process, termed *luteinisation*, occurs under the influence of luteinising hormone (LH) and prolactin, the two major luteotrophic hormones in rodents. Luteinisation is accompanied by degeneration of the basement membrane separating the theca interna and zona granulosa, and infiltration of the postovulatory follicle by blood vessels from the theca interna. The resulting mature *corpus luteum* ("yellow body") is a large eosinophilic structure that may bulge out from the ovarian surface or obscure the ovarian corticomedullary junction, depending on its location. Note that prior to luteinisation immature corpora lutea typically appear more basophilic .

Formation of Corpus albicans

Each corpus luteum matures during the oestrous cycle in which it is formed before regressing over the course of several subsequent cycles. Consequently, at least three sets of corpora lutea are present within the ovaries of normally cycling rats. Degenerating corpora lutea progressively shrink in size and are characterised by increased amounts of fibrous tissue and yellow-brown lipofuscin pigment . The fibrous tissue mass that constitutes the corpus luteum during the final stages of regression is termed the *corpus albicans* ("white body"). In the rat this structure undergoes complete regression and leaves no fibrous tissue remnant within the ovary.

Ultrastructure of Corpus luteum

There was no obvious luteal ultrastructural difference between new CL and old CL at the diestrus stage in the control group. During the diestrus stage, lipid droplets, smooth and rough endoplasmic reticulum (SER and RER, respectively), and mitochondria were uniformly distributed in the luteal cells of the control rats .

Histology and Ultrastructure of the Regressing Corpus Luteum

Histologic evidence of regression includes shrinkage of cells in the granulosa layer. Theca and granulosa cells are progressively vacuolized, accounting in the former for the distinctive appearance of so-called mulberry cells. Histochemical studies show rapid loss of key steroidogenic enzymes. Ultrastructurally, there is breakdown of the organization of the endoplasmic reticulum, Golgi regression, and appearance of lipid droplet inclusions. The lutein zone exhibits progressive fibrosis, which presages ultimate hyalinization. Connective tissue organization of the central cavity continues, but even in the latest specimens fresh hemorrhage often is encountered.

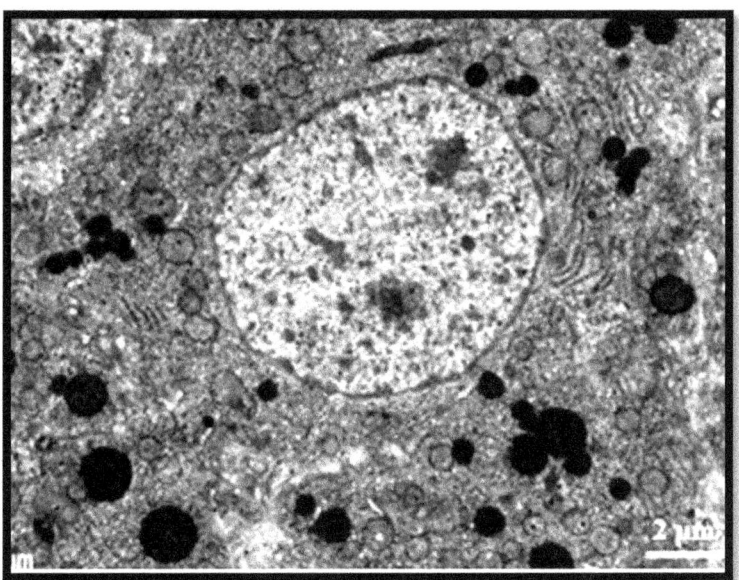

Fig. 41. Ultrastructural luteal changes in the control rat and formation of new CL(corpus luteum) at the diestrus stage. Magnification 8,000 X.

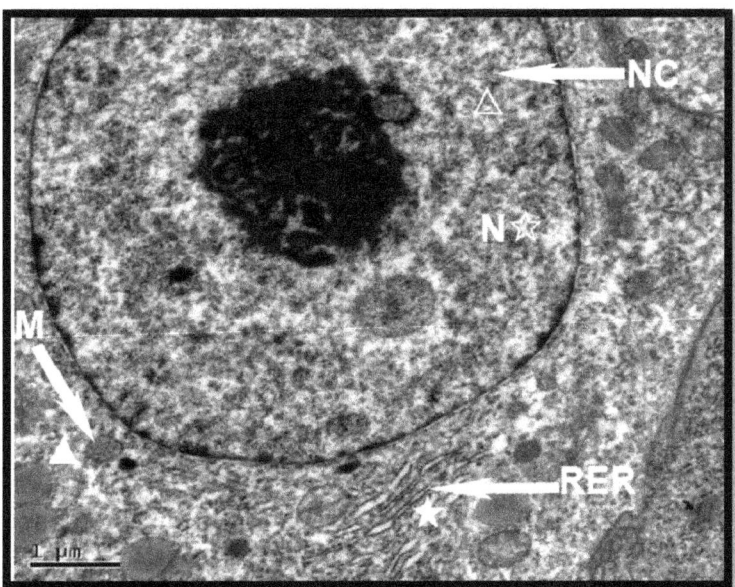

Fig. 42. The ultrastructural changes of the rats' ovarian tissues were observed by transmission electron microscopy, A) A representative rat's ovarian tissue section from the control group, which had normal appearance (X10000).
M: mitochondria, N: nucleus, RER: rough endoplasmic reticulum, NC: nuclear chromatin, MC: mitochondrial cristae.

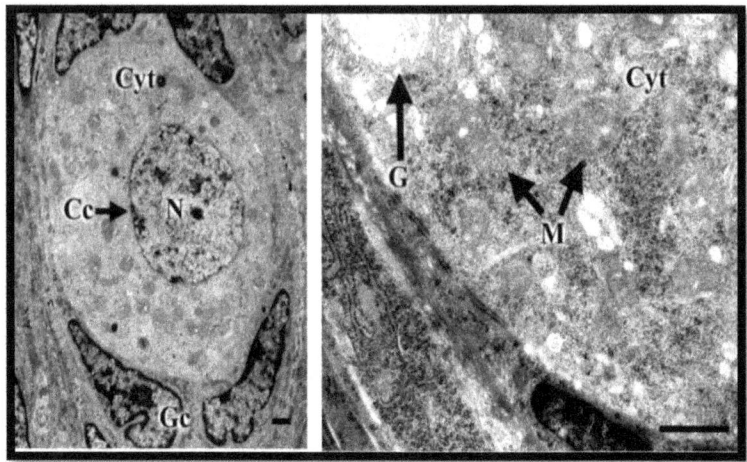

Fig. 43. Healthy and atretic rat ovarian primordial follicles. Representative electron photomicrographs of A) a healthy primordial rat ovarian follicle, demonstrating the appearance of the cytoplasm (Cyt) and nucleus (N), containing small amounts of condensed chromatin (Cc), of the oocyte and surrounding granulosa cells (Gc); B) oocyte cytoplasm containing faintly staining healthy mitochondria (M) with shelflike cristae and Golgi apparatus(G). Bars = 1 µm. Original magnifications were A) x 8100, B) x14 000,

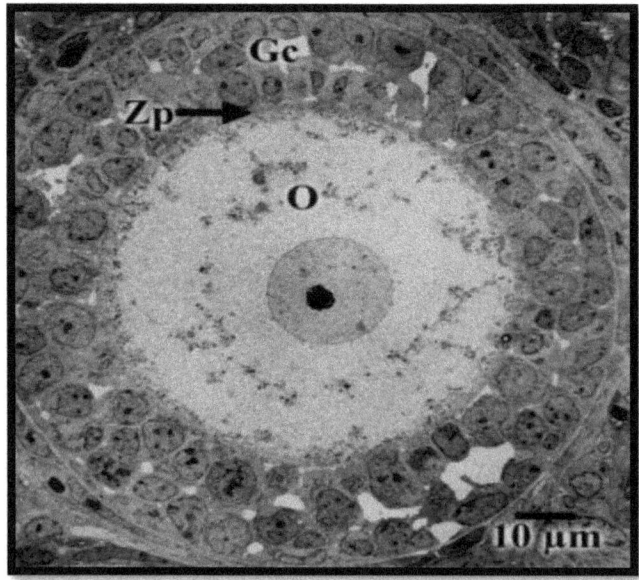

Fig. 44. Healthy rat ovarian preantral follicle. Electron photomicrographs showing the appearance of A) a healthy growing rat ovarian follicle containing two layers of granulosa cells (Gc) and the zona pellucida (Zp) surrounding the oocyte (O) ; Original magnifications were A) X 1570.

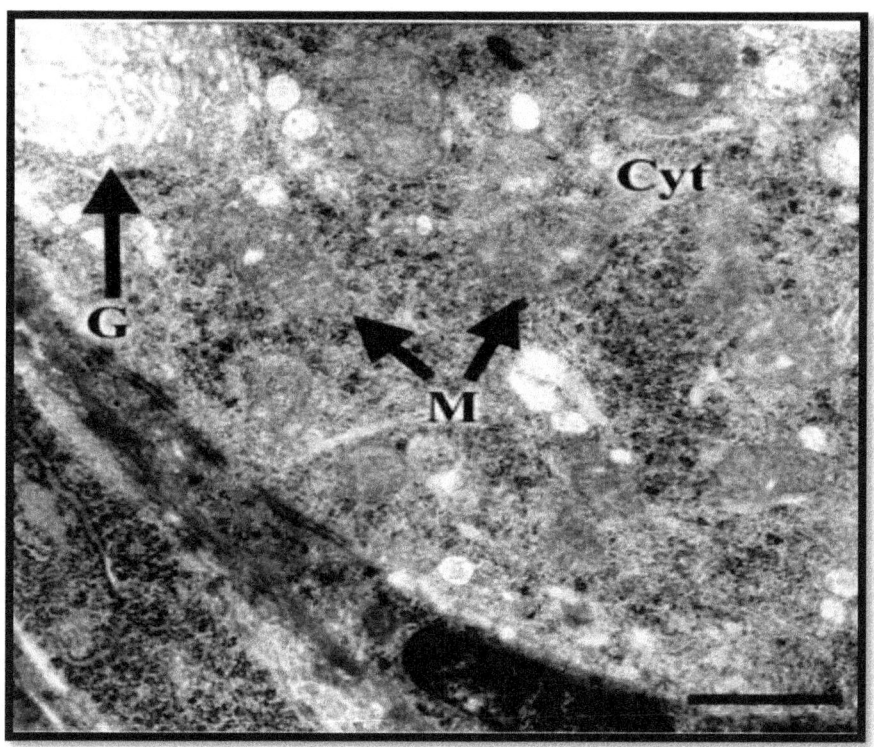

Fig. 45. Oocyte cytoplasm containing faintly staining healthy mitochondria (M) with shelflike cristae and Golgi apparatus (G); Original magnifications were X14000.

CONTRIBUTION OF SCIENTISTS

Reinier de Graaf

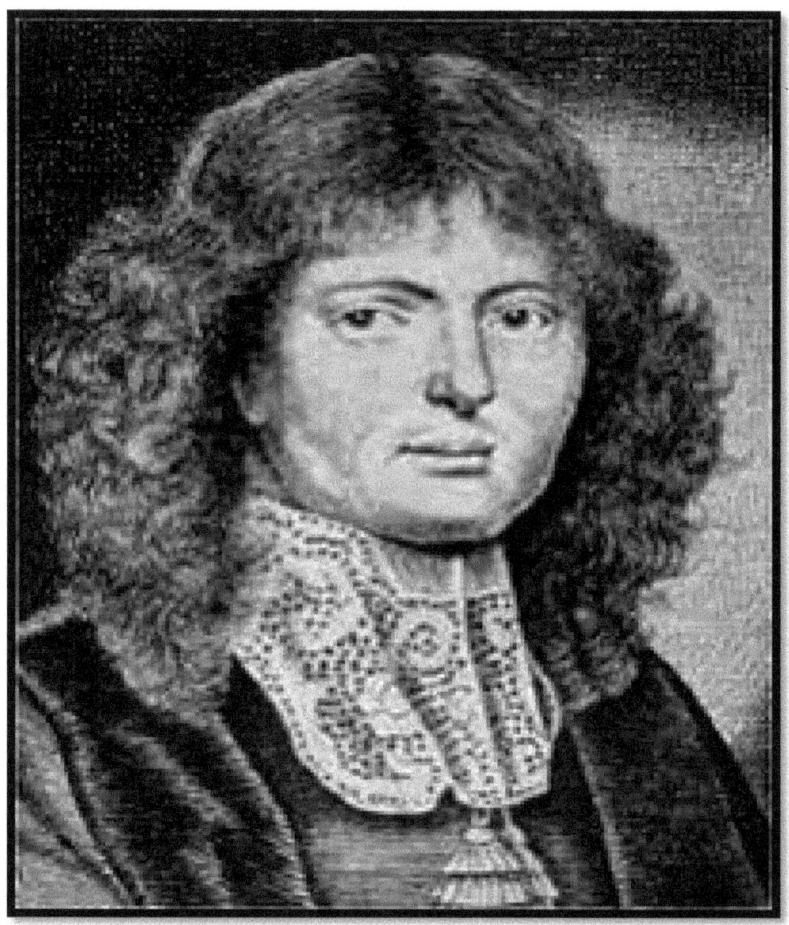

Reinier de Graaf

Born: July 30, 1641 Netherlands

Died: August 17, 1673 (aged 32) Delft Netherlands

Subjects Of Study: mammal; human reproductive system; ovarian follicle; pancreas

Contribution

Regnier de Graaf (1641-1673)

Regnier de Graaf, a Dutch physician and anatomist, was born 30 July 1641 in Schoonhoven, the Netherlands. Though he published papers on both pancreatic and male reproductive anatomy, he is best known for his discovery of the mature ovarian follicles as well as his contributions to the general body of knowledge surrounding the female mammalian reproductive organs.

THE THYROID GLAND

ANATOMY OF THE THYROID GLAND

The thyroid gland is located in the anterior neck and spans the C5-T1 vertebrae. It consists of two lobes (left and right), which are connected by a central isthmus anteriorly – this produces a butterfly-shape appearance.

The lobes of the thyroid gland are wrapped around the cricoid cartilage and superior rings of the trachea. The gland is located within the visceral compartment of the neck (along with the trachea, oesophagus and pharynx). This compartment is bound by the pretracheal fascia.

Blood supply

The thyroid gland is highly vascularised. The arterial supply to the thyroid gland is via two main arteries: Superior thyroid artery and Inferior thyroid artery . The Venous drainage is carried by the superior, middle, and inferior thyroid veins, which form a venous plexus around the thyroid gland.

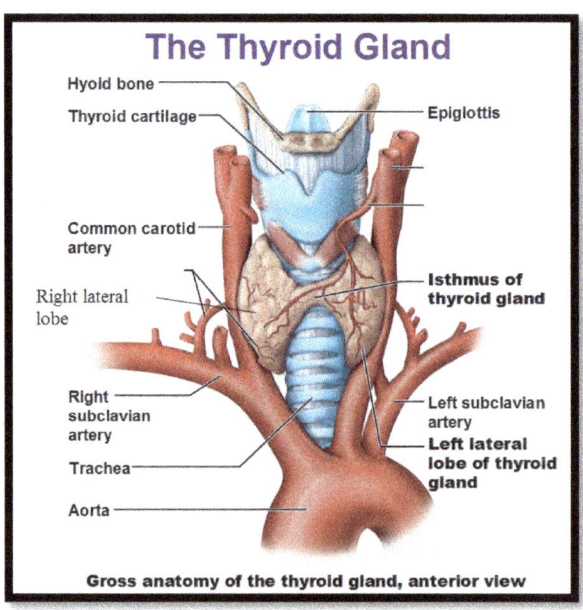

Fig. 46. Anatomical position of the thyroid gland in rat

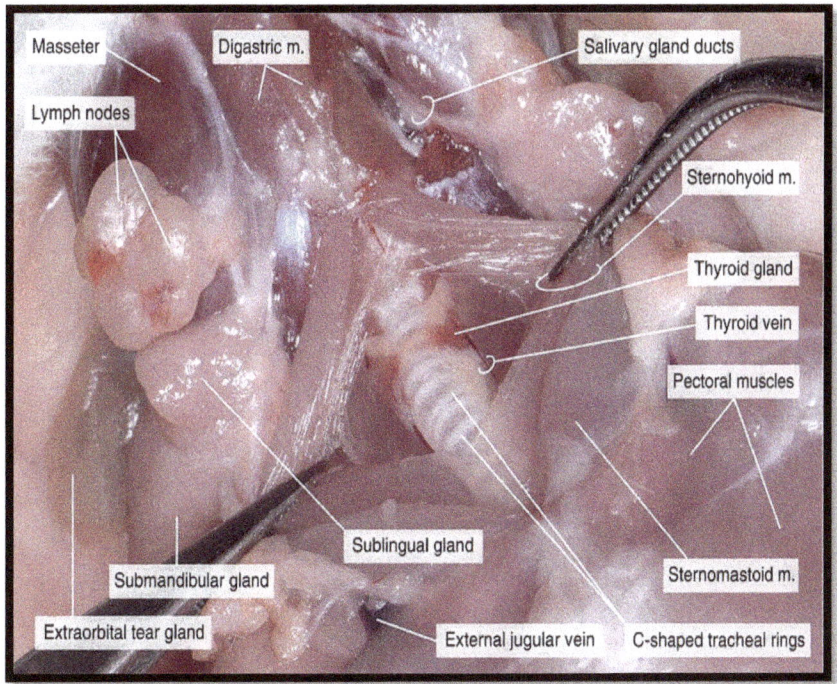

Fig. 47. Rat dissection (*Rattus norvegicus*) : Exact location of the thyroid gland

Anatomical position

In most mammals the thyroid gland is located caudal to the trachea at the level of the first or second tracheal ring. The thyroid gland is composed of two lobes lying on either side of the trachea and connected by a narrow piece of tissue called the **isthmus.**

Histological structures of the Thyroid gland

Histological Structure

The thyroid gland is divided into lobules by the septae dipping from the capsule. The thyroid lobules consist of a large number of typical units called thyroid follicles. The thyroid follicles are the structural and functional units of a thyroid gland. These are spherical, and the wall is made up of a large number of cuboidal cells, the follicular cells. These follicular cells are the derivates of the endoderm and secrete thyroid hormone. The circulating form of this hormone is thyroxine, which is tetraiodothyronine (T4) along with a small quantity of triiodothyronine (T3). Even though most of T4 later converts to the more active form T3, both affect the target cells with varying degrees of stimulation. These hormones help in regulating the BMR of the body. In between these thyroid follicles or within the wall of the thyroid follicles, we find the small C cells, also know as Parafollicular cells. These are derived from neural crest cells and secrete polypeptide hormone known as calcitonin. The calcitonin helps in depositing calcium and phosphate in skeletal and other tissues leading to hypocalcemia. This function is the opposite of the parathormone.

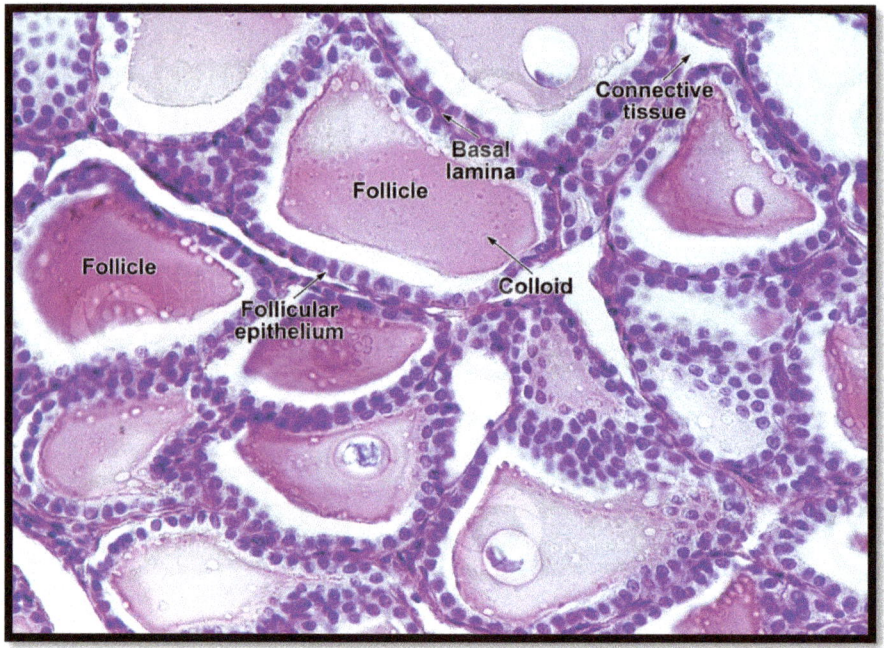

Fig. 48. Histological structure of the Rat thyroid gland. 400x.
F: Follicle ; C : Colloid ; Conn. : Connective tissue ; B : Basal lamina ; F : Follicular epithelium

Ultrastructure

Ultrastructurally, the thyroid follicular cell exhibits numerous microvilli on its luminal surface, particularly during active resorption . The cell membranes of adjacent cells interdigitate in a complex fashion and are joined by a junctional complex toward the apex. At the base, a continuous basal lamina separates the follicular cell from the stroma. The cytoplasm contains an abundant granular endoplasmic reticulum and a well-developed Golgi apparatus. The latter is located between the nucleus and the luminal surface, and becomes prominent in actively secreting cells. the follicular cells of the control rats had euchromatic nuclei, intact lysosomes and endoplasmic reticulum. Mitochondria are well represented; their length and cytoplasmic location vary according to the functional status of the cell. Lysosomes are numerous in actively secreting cells; most are located toward the apical side.

The parafollicular cells of the control rats had large euchromatic nuclei. In addition to the mitochondria, endoplasmic reticulum and lysosomes, the cytoplasm contained electron dense granules.

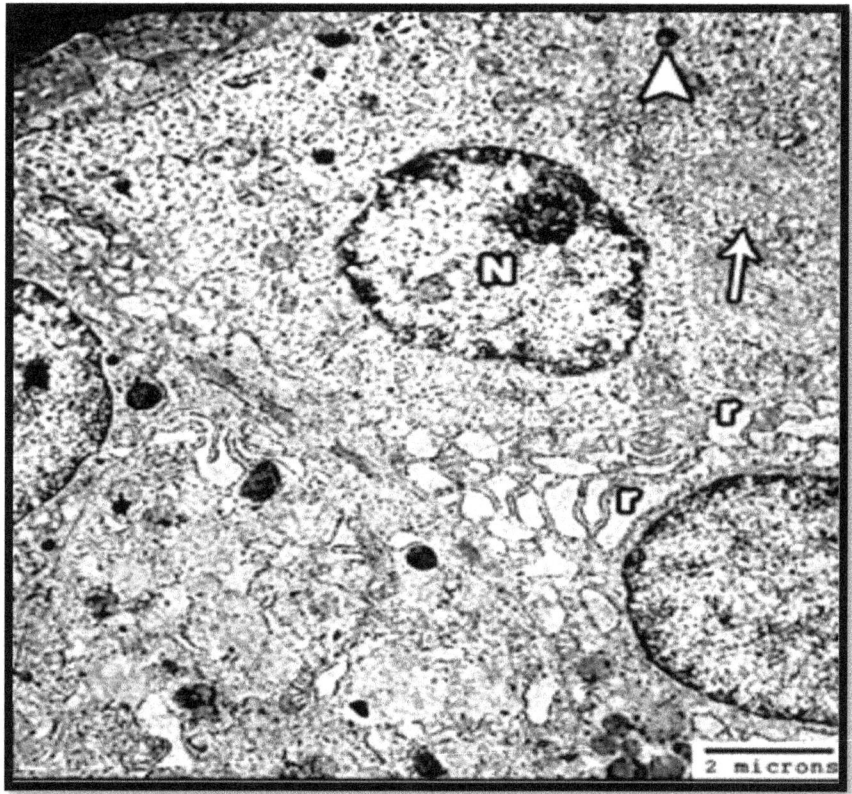

Fig. 49. (A) Thyroid gland of control rat showing follicular cells with euchromatic nuclei (N), lysosomes (arrow head) and endoplasmic reticulum (r).

CONTRIBUTION OF SCIENTIST ON THYROID GLAND FUNCTION

EMIL THEODOR KOCHER

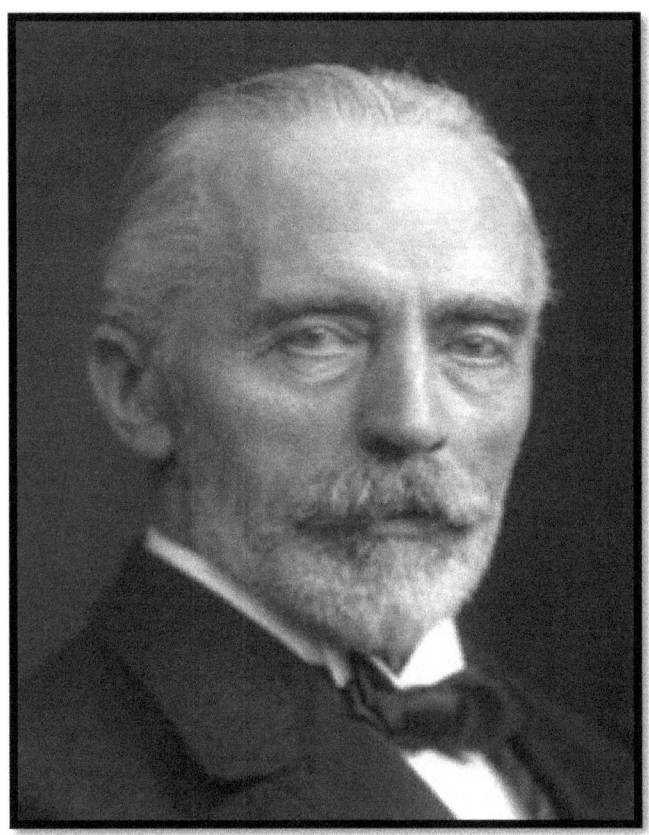

EMIL THEODOR KOCHER

The Nobel Prize in Physiology or Medicine 1909

Born: 25 August 1841, Berne, Switzerland

Died: 27 July 1917, Berne, Switzerland

Affiliation at the time of the award: Berne University, Berne, Switzerland

Work

The thyroid gland is a gland in the neck that is destroyed by goiters, which can lead to difficulty in breathing in serious cases. This led to attempts to remove the gland by surgery. However, this was risky and could result in serious health problems. In 1883 Theodor Kocher shed light on the thyroid gland's function in metabolism, among other things, and showed how surgery could be carried out more safely through good hygiene and minimal blood loss. He also showed that a viable part of the gland needs to be left intact during the operation.

Parathyroid gland

Anatomical position of the Parathyroid gland

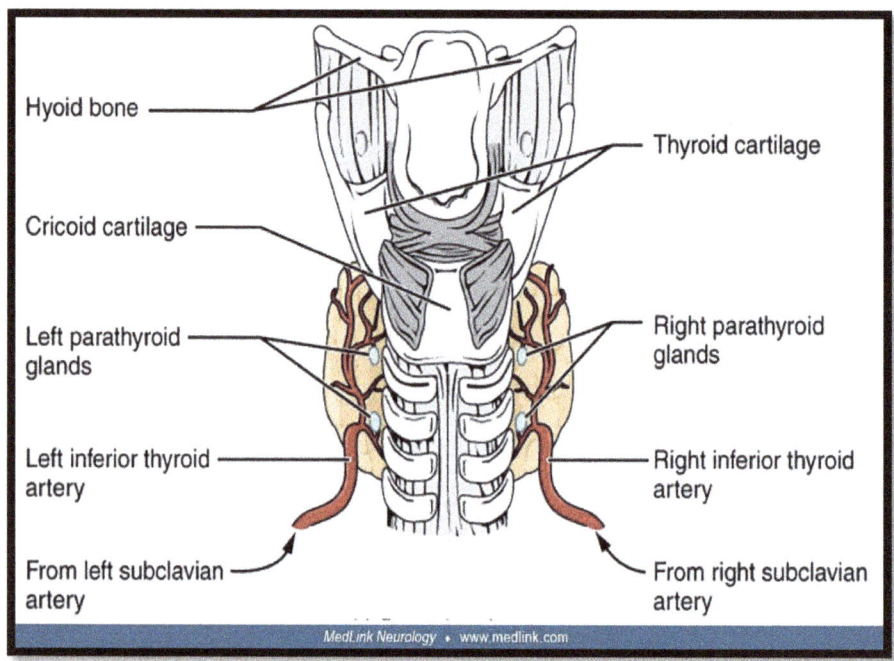

Fig. 50. Anatomical position of the thyroid and parathyroid gland

Anatomical position of the Parathyroid gland

The parathyroid glands are tiny, round structures usually found embedded in the posterior surface of the thyroid gland . A thick connective tissue capsule separates the glands from the thyroid tissue. Usually four parathyroid glands are present , but occasionally there are more in tissues of the neck or chest. The function of one type of parathyroid cells, the oxyphil cells, is not clear. The primary functional cells of the parathyroid glands are the chief cells. These epithelial cells produce and secrete the parathyroid hormone (PTH), the major hormone involved in the regulation of blood calcium levels.

Vasculature

The vascular supply is similar to that of the thyroid gland. Arterial supply is chiefly via the inferior thyroid artery (as this artery supplies the posterior aspect of the thyroid gland – where the parathyroids are located). Collateral arterial supply is from the superior thyroid artery and thyroid ima artery.

Venous drainage is into the superior, middle, and inferior thyroid veins.

Histological structures

Histologically, the parathyroid glands are bounded by a thin connective tissue capsule that overlies a network of adipose tissue, blood vessels and glandular parenchyma. The amount of stromal fibro adipose tissue increases with aging, eventually comprising approximately 50% of the gland volume in elderly. Connective tissue septa separate gland into small irregular lobules, that contain mainly densely packed dense cords of cells clustered around capillaries. The parenchymal cells of the parathyroid gland of control animals are classified under a microscope into two main types of cells : chief cells and oxyphil cells.

Principal (chief) cells are the more numerous of the parenchymal cells of the parathyroid.

Chief cells are small, polygonal cells, with a centrally located nucleus of rounded shape. The cytoplasm of the chief cells has typical organelles that are involved in protein synthesis.

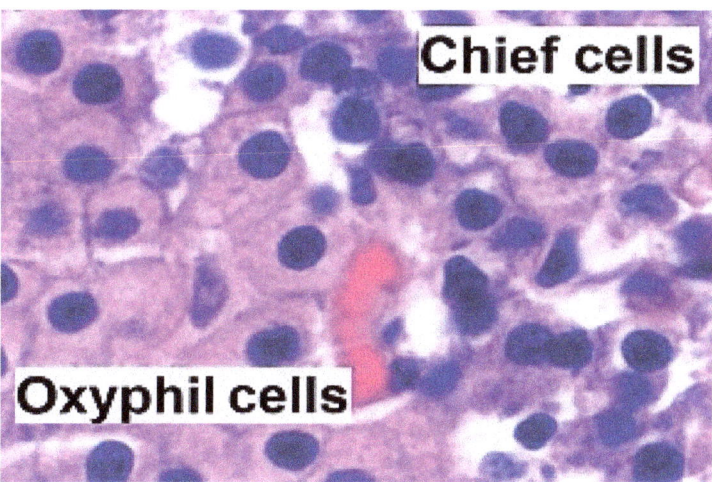

Fig. 51. High magnification micrograph. H&E stain. The small, dark cells are chief cells, which are responsible for secreting parathyroid hormone. The cells with orange/pink staining cytoplasm are oxyphil cells . 1000x

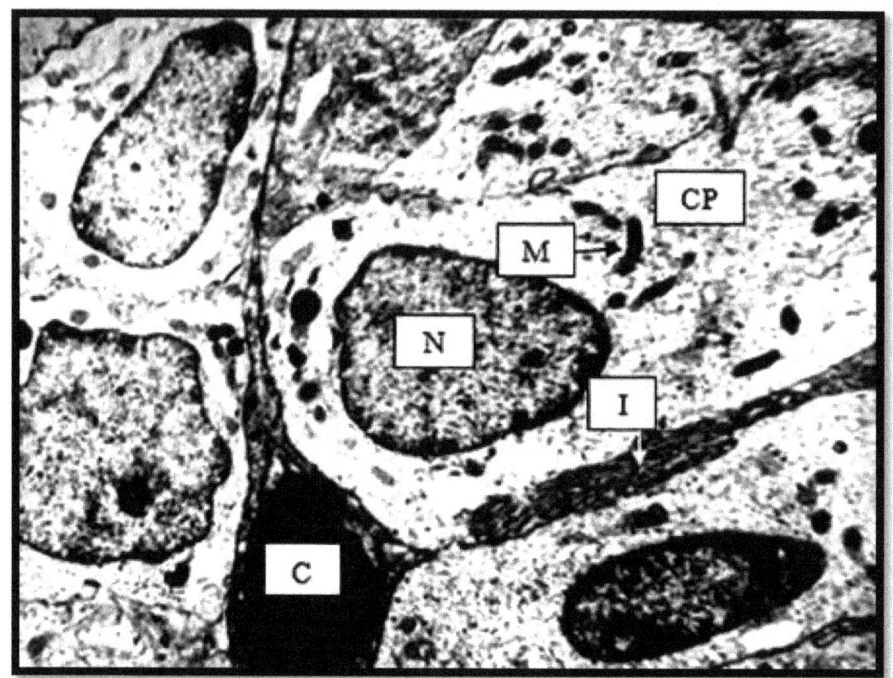

Fig. 52. Parathyroid gland of the intact rat. TEM. Magnification X8000.
CP- chief parathyrocyte, N – nucleus, I – interdigitation, M – mitochondria, C – blood capillary.

Histological Structures of the Parathyroid gland :

Histologically, the parathyroid glands are bounded by a thin connective tissue capsule that overlies a network of adipose tissue, blood vessels and glandular parenchyma. The amount of stromal fibro adipose tissue increases with aging, eventually comprising approximately 50% of the gland volume in elderly. Connective tissue septa separate gland into small irregular lobules, that contain mainly densely packed dense cords of cells clustered around capillaries. The parenchymal cells of the parathyroid gland of control animals are classified into two main types of cells : chief cells and oxyphil cells. Principal (chief) cells are more numerous of the parenchymal cells of the parathyroid.

Chief cells

Chief cells are small, polygonal cells, with a centrally located nucleus of rounded shape.

The cytoplasm of the chief cells has typical organelles that are involved in protein synthesis. Depending on the stages of secretory cycle, all chief cells could be classified into inactive and active types. The cytoplasm of inactive light cells contains poorly developed synthetic organelles and infrequent secretory granules. There are numerous lipid droplets, lysosomes or glycogen inclusions. Lysosomes differ from secretory granules in larger sizes and high electron density.

Dark chief cells, that represent the active stage of the secretory cycle, are oval or polygonal in shape. The plasma membranes of adjacent chief cells have a tortuous course, which is justified by the presence of complex interdigitations. The nuclei are oval or spherical, with occasional shallow invaginations. The cells have rich free ribosomes and a rough endoplasmic reticulum. The Golgi complexes contain numerous prosecretory granules. The secretory granules of different sizes are located around the Golgi complexes and peripheral cytoplasm. Some of them are situated close to the plasma membrane.

Oxyphil cells

Oxyphil cells constitute a minor portion of the parenchymal cells. Their cells are larger, stain darker, and are much fewer than chief cells. Oxyphil cells appear in small rare clusters, and their function is unknown, although some investigators suggest that they are inactive chief cells. The key morphological difference of this type is the abundant cytoplasm filled with numerous large mitochondria. The rough endoplasmic reticulum is scarce and the Golgi complex associated with few prosecretory granules is poorly developed. A few secretory granules, lysosomes, lipid droplets and glycogen particles are present.

N.B.: Chief cells play a central role in calcium homeostasis, by releasing the appropriate amount of parathyroid hormone to correct or maintain normal blood calcium levels. When blood calcium levels decrease, the parathyroid glands secrete parathormone (PTH), activating osteoblasts to secrete osteoclast-stimulating factor and to suppress bone formation. As a result, dormant osteoclasts are activated, and the formation of new osteoclasts is induced, initiating bone resorption and ultimately leading to calcium ions being released from the bone and transferred to the bloodstream.

Ultrastructural Evaluation of the Parathyroid Gland

In the control groups, the chief cells were oval or polygonal in shape. The nucleus was irregularly shaped, having a few spots of chromatin area located in the margin, and the nuclear membrane was infolded. The plasma membrane showed interdigitations of the tortuous plasma membranes and the intercellular spaces were narrow. Free ribosomes were diffusely scattered in the cytoplasm. Mitochondria were dispersed throughout the cytoplasm, the cisternae of the rough-surfaced endoplasmic reticulum (rER) were arranged in parallel arrays or randomly distributed in the cytoplasm, and the Golgi complexes were well developed and contained a few coated vesicles and numerous prosecretory granules. Storage granules, 300–620 nm in diameter, were filled with a finely particulate and an electron-dense material, and were scattered in the Golgi area as well as in the cytoplasm . Lipid droplets were occasionally present in the cytoplasm (Isono et al., 1990; Chen et al., 2001).

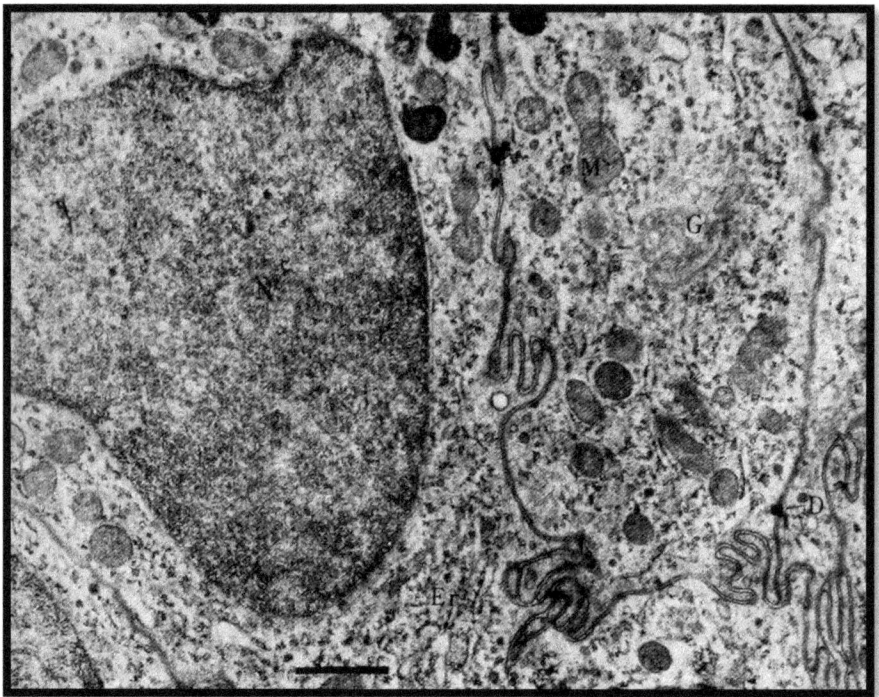

Fig. 53. The dark principal cell has many complicated interdigitations with desmosomes (D). It has many free ribosomes, mitochondria (M), Golgi apparatus (G) and endoplasmic reticulum (Er). Golgi apparatus is surrounded with small vesicles of varying electron density. The nucleus (N) is ovoid and irregular in outline.

CONTRIBUTION OF SCIENTIST ON PARATHYROID GLAND FUNCTION

James Bertram Collip

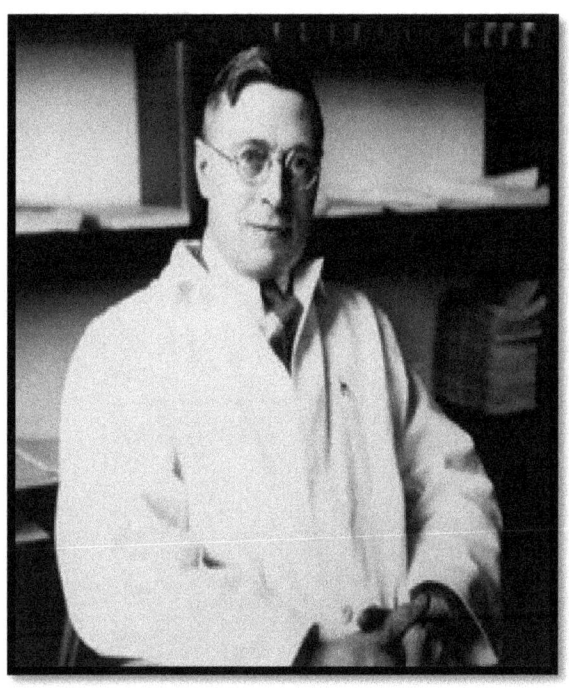

James Bertram Collip
Born: James Bertram Collip November 20, 1892 Belleville, Ontario
Died: June 19, 1965 (aged 72) London, Ontario
Citizenship: Canadian
Alma mater: University of Toronto
Known for: Insulin

Major Contribution of Professor Collip

James Collip was a biochemist who proved vital in producing the first insulin dose that was suitable for use on humans.

In 1921, Collip took a sabbatical from the University of Alberta and worked with Frederick Banting and Charles Best at the University of Toronto. He had previously received his PhD in biochemistry in 1916.

Banting and Best had discovered insulin, but the extract was raw and after being administered to Leonard Thompson, the first human to receive it, no changes were seen in his diabetic condition.

Collip purified this extract within two weeks and it was again administered to Thompson. This time, the insulin led to Thompson's blood glucose levels stabilising, which saved his life.

Collip received a quarter of the prize money awarded to Banting as part of the Nobel Prize in 1923, and despite enduring many arguments with Banting during the discovery of insulin, the two became good friends in the 1930s.

In 1928, Collip became the Professor of Biochemistry at McGill University, while he later served as the Dean of Medicine at the University of Western Ontario between 1947 and 1961.

Collip plunged into endocrinological research and was one of the first to isolate the parathyroid hormone. In 1928 he succeeded Archibald Byron Macallum as professor of biochemistry at McGill University, where for the next decade he and his students were leaders in endocrinology, pioneering in the isolation and study of the ovarian and gonadotrophic hormones.

THYMUS GLAND

Anatomical position of the Thymus gland

The thymus gland is a pink, lobulated lymphoid organ, located in the thoracic cavity and neck. In the adolescent, it is involved the development of the immune system. After puberty, it decreases in size and is slowly replaced by fat. The lobules are comprised of a series of follicles, which have a medullary and cortical component.

The gland is mainly located within the thoracic superior mediastinum, posterior to the manubrium of the sternum. However, in some individuals, it can extend superiorly into the neck (reaching the thyroid gland), and inferiorly into the anterior mediastinum (lying in front of the fibrous pericardium).

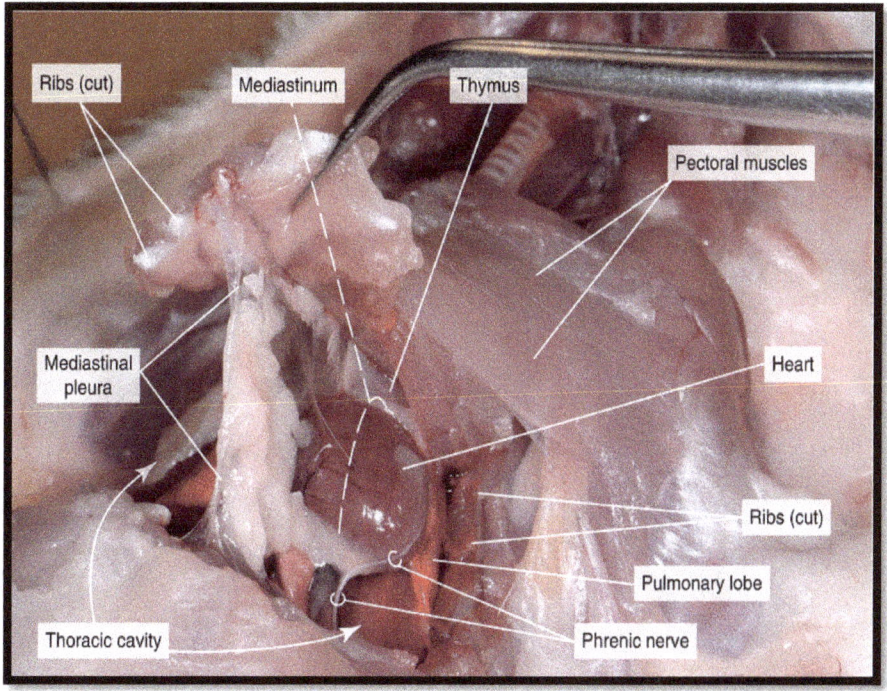

Fig. 54. Position of the Thymus gland in *Rattus* sp.(from the dissected animal)

Histological structure

The thymus gland is a pink, lobulated lymphoid organ, located in the thoracic cavity and neck. Both lobes of the thymus are enclosed by an outer layer of the capsule and divided into lob ules by septa which extend from the inner layer of the capsule to the corticomedullary junction. The septa form an irregular network. As a consequence, the lobules are variable in shape, size, and orientation. From the capsule and septa, trabeculae spread through the cortex to the medulla. The medulla was less densely cellular than the cortex, with many epithelial reticular cells and Hassall's corpuscles. The cortex and medulla were separated by a highly vascular corticomedullary zone.

The thymic cortex had many pale stained areas. These pale areas showed lymphocytic depletion with the exposure of epithelial reticular cells. Many lymphocytes were shrunk with pyknotic nuclei. Many degenerated thymic epithelial reticular cells appeared in the medulla.

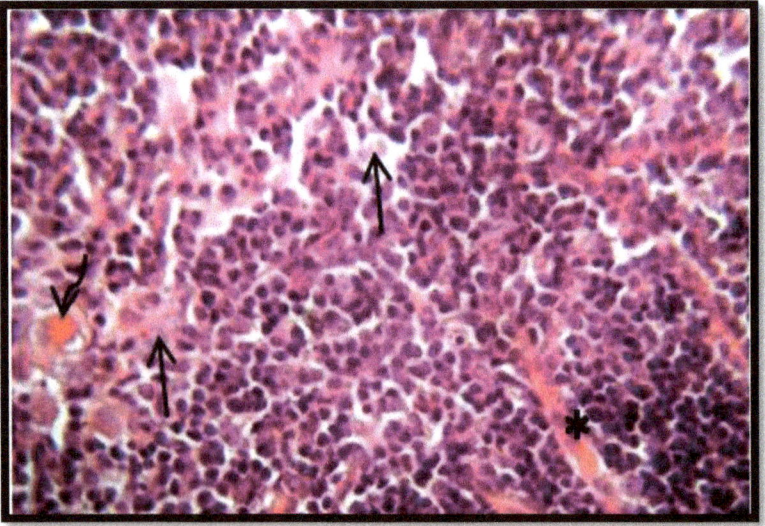

Fig. 55. Higher magnification of the thymic medulla showing less cellular density than the cortex, and contains more prominent epithelial cells (arrow) and Hassalls corpuscles (curved arrow). Notice plentiful blood vessels at the corticomedullary junction (*). X 400 (H& E).

Cells of the Thymus

Inside the thymus gland, there are many different cells. These include:[2]
- Epithelial cells line all body surfaces and act as a protective barrier.

- Kulchitsky cells make hormones, chemical messengers for the thymus and other cells.
- Thymocytes are cells that become mature T lymphocytes, specialized infection fighters.
- Dendritic cells are found in the skin and other tissues. They help protect against toxins and other foreign substances.
- Macrophages are cells that are sometimes called the "garbage trucks" of the immune system. They eat foreign matter and clear away tumors.
- B lymphocytes are cells that make antibodies, proteins that attack viruses and bacteria.
- Myoid cells are muscle-like cells. Scientists believe they trigger the autoimmune response in a muscle disorder.

This list hints at how complex the thymus gland's job is. Its role also changes throughout your life.

Hormone Production

The thymus gland produces **several hormones**, including:
- Thymopoietin and thymulin: These hormones are involved in the process where T cells get turned into different types of disease fighters.
- Thymosin: This hormone boosts the immune system's response. Thymosin also stimulates hormones that control growth.
- Thymic humoral factor: These hormones increase the immune system's response to viruses.

The thymus gland also makes small amounts of hormones produced in other areas of the body. These include **melatonin,** which helps you sleep, and **insulin**, which helps control your **blood sugar**.

The fine structure of thymic cortical epithelium of normal rats

The fine structure of the thymic cortex from control groups was similar to that described previously in various mammalian species. The epithelial cells were easily identified by the presence of tonofilaments and desmosomes, which are the two specific characteristics of thymic epithelial cells. TCE were spidery in shape with long cytoplasmic processes extending in various directions and bordering the connective septae, the vessels and the thymocytes in a more or less sparse and continuous anastomosed network. The large nucleus had a clear, dispersed chromatin which was more euchromatic than that of surrounding thymocytes and also had a thin rim of heterochromatin along the nuclear envelope (Figs. 1, 2). The nucleolus was prominent and reticulated. The cytoplasm contained vacuoles, dense bundles of tonofilaments and relatively sparse cellular organelles . The vacuoles were generally electron-lucent, but contained granular electron-dense material located mainly near their limiting membranes. Sometimes, the vacuoles also contained small empty vesicles . As a rule, the Golgi apparatus and rough endoplasmic reticulum (RER) were rather poorly developed . There were several mitochondria and a few free ribosomes scattered throughout the cytoplasm.

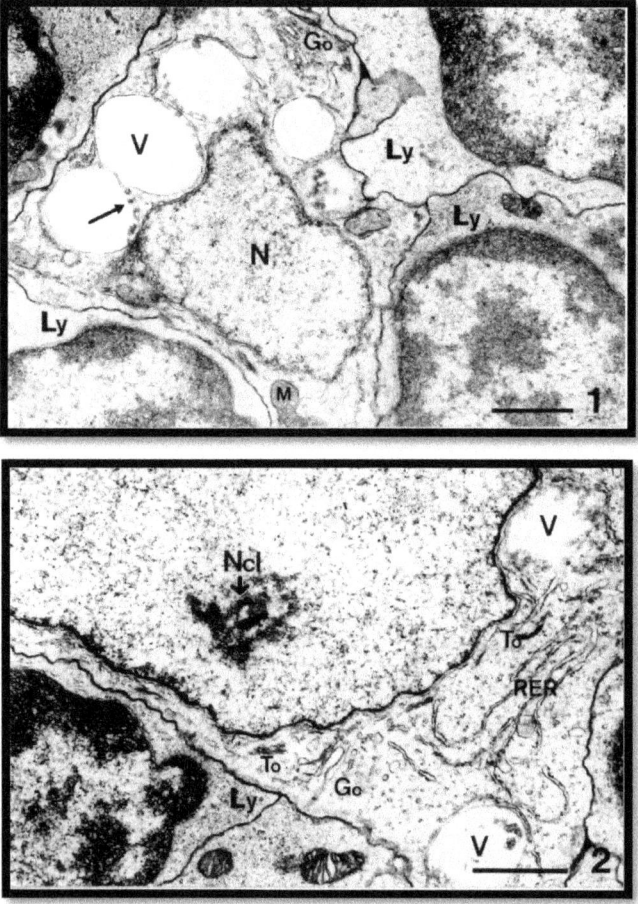

Fig. 56 1 and 2. Normal rat thymic cortex %. The thymic cortical epithelial cells are characterized by tonofilaments (To), a prominent nucleus (N) and a nucleolus (Ncl) as well as large electron-lucent vacuoles (V) containing electron dense granular material along their inner espect of the limiting mernbranes (arrow). M: rnitochondria; RER: rough endoplasmic reticulum; Go: Golgi apparatus; Ly: lymphocytes. Bar: 1 µm

Contribution of Scientist

Professor Jacques Miller

Emeritus Professor Jacques Miller AC from Melbourne's Walter and Eliza Hall Institute has won a Lasker Award, one of the highest international honours in medical research.

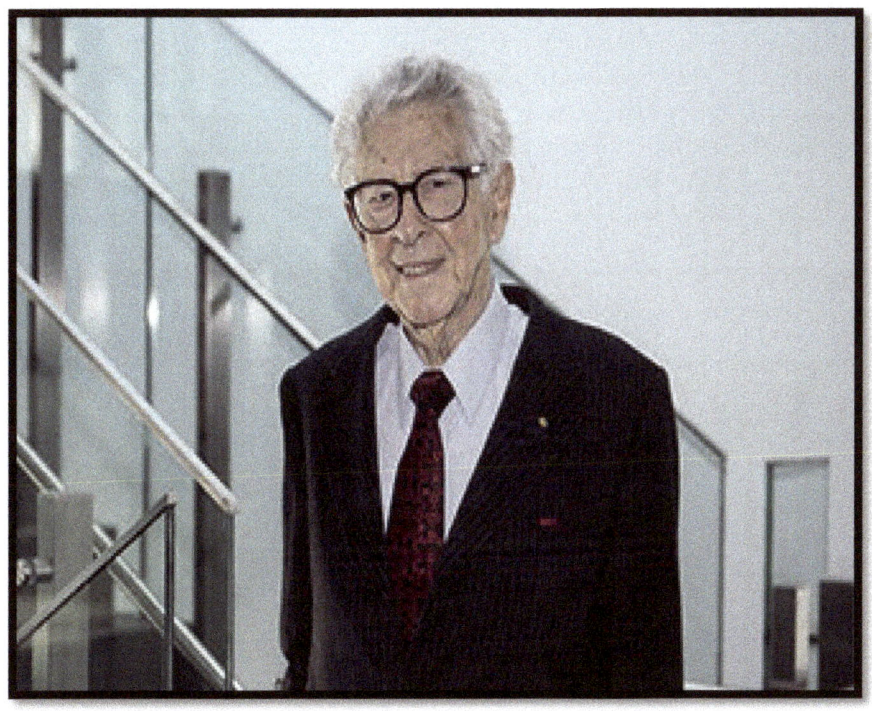

Jacques Francis Albert Pierre Miller AC FRS FAA (born 2 April 1931) is a French-Australian research scientist. He is known for having discovered the function of the thymus and for the identification, in mammalian species of the two major subsets of lymphocytes (T cells and B cells) and their function.

Professor Miller was joint recipient of the 2019 Albert Lasker Basic Medical Research Award with Professor Max Cooper of Emory University, US. They received the award for identifying immune cells called T and B cells, which have critical roles in our immune system.

The impact of this discovery on modern medicine is immense, and underpins many important innovations including vaccine development, organ transplants, identifying and treating autoimmune diseases and immunotherapy to treat cancer.

KIDNEY

Anatomical Position of the Kidney

The kidneys of the albino rats were bean – shaped, smooth, reddish-brown color were covered by a thin connective tissue capsule that was adherent to sub capsular connective tissue occasional fibroblast. The rat kidneys lay alongside the vertebral column in the abdominal cavity , the right kidney was situated more cranially than the left kidney. Renal arteries and veins supply the kidneys with blood.

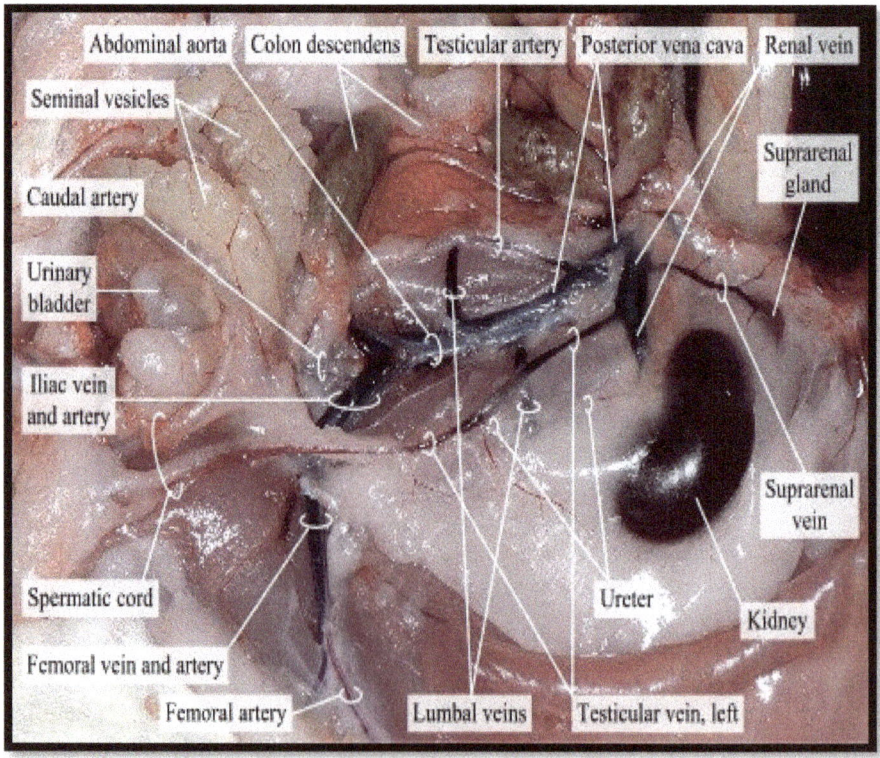

Fig. 57. Anatomical position of the kidney (from dissected specimen)

Histological structures of the Kidney :

The rat kidneys were reddish-brown color were covered by a thin connective tissue capsule . The kidney has a typical bean-shaped appearance . It consists of superficial capsule, outer cortex and inner medulla. The outer cortex is highly vascular; the inner medulla is slightly thick and less vascular. Both cortex and medulla are built up of different tubule structures. The nephron is the functional unit of the kidney; each nephron consists of corpuscle, proximal convoluted tubules, loop of Henle, distal convoluted tubules and collecting tubules. Bowman's capsule is formed of two thin cellular layers, an inner visceral layer and an outer parietal one, which is a simple squamous epithelium resting on basal lamina. The visceral layer is formed of flattened epithelium.

Kidney Tissue (Control)

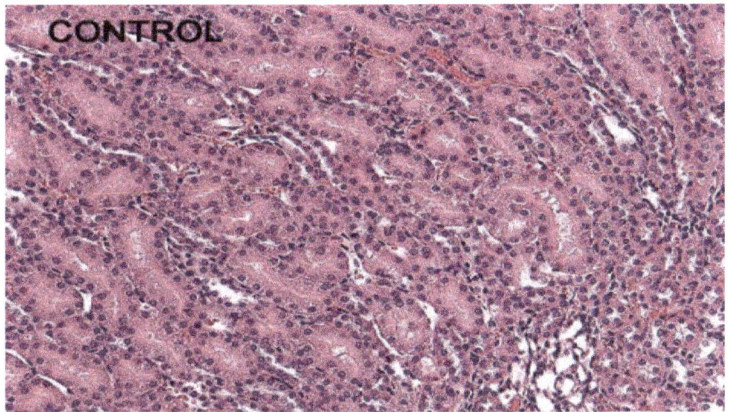

Fig. 58. Kidney morphology (×20 magnification) of control

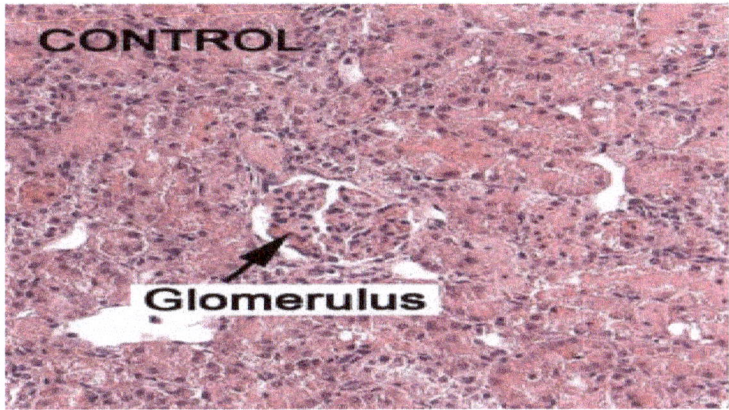

Fig. 59. Morphology of rat kidney slices of control Magnification is ×20.

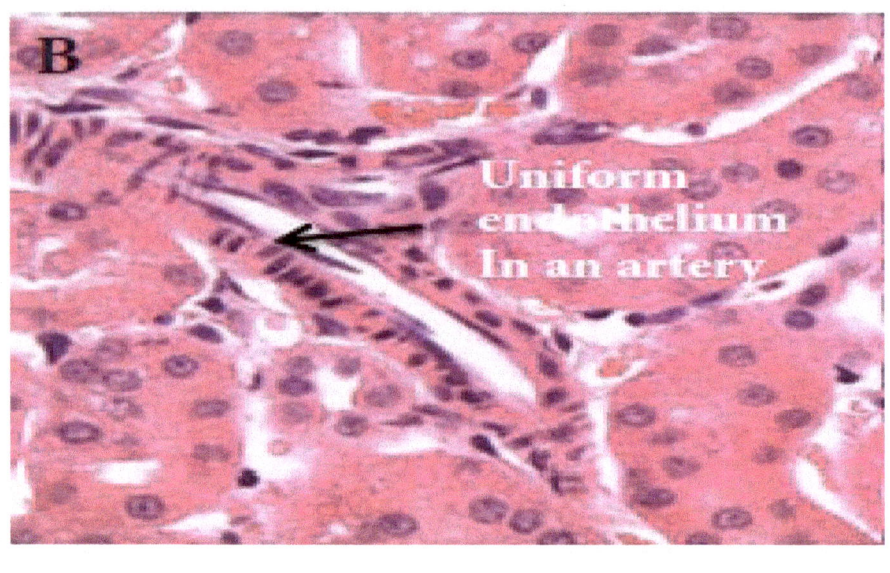

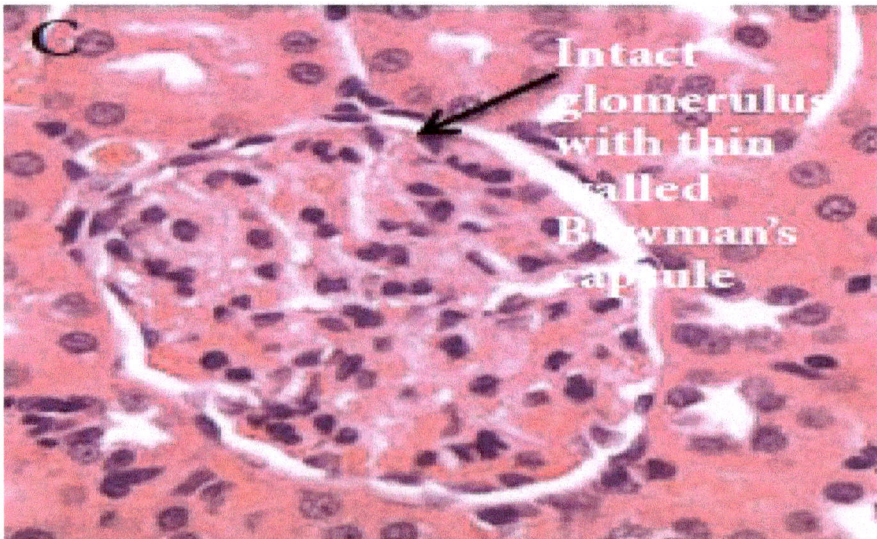

Fig. 60 b and c. Histological images of rat renal cortex sections. Renal cortex H&E (x400) paraffin sections .

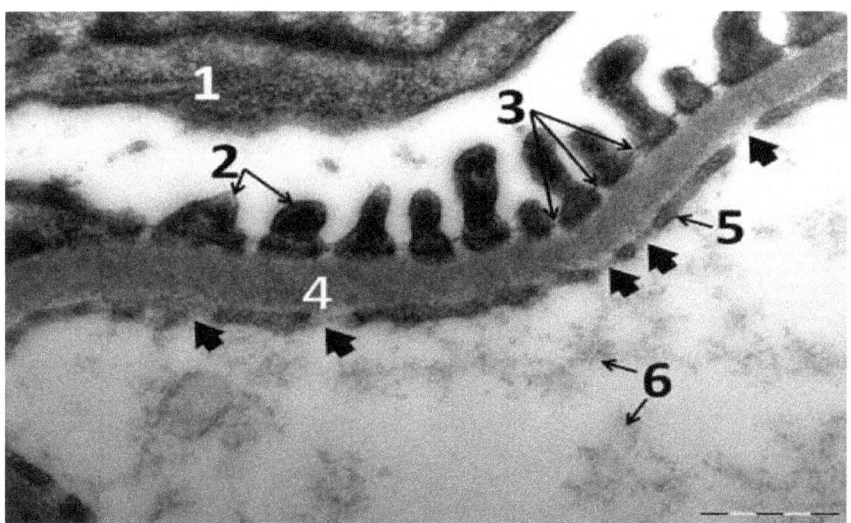

Fig. 61. Electron micrograph of the rat glomerulus, control (healthy) kidney. 1 – body of the podocyte; 2 – numerous pedicles of podocytes abutting the glomerular basement membrane (GBM); 3 – diaphragm between the pedicles of podocytes ; 4 – GBM without thickening ; 5 – fenestrated endothelia (arrowheads); 6 – precipitated plasma proteins. Lead citrate and uranyl acetate (Pb Citrate +UA); orig. magn. 28000x.

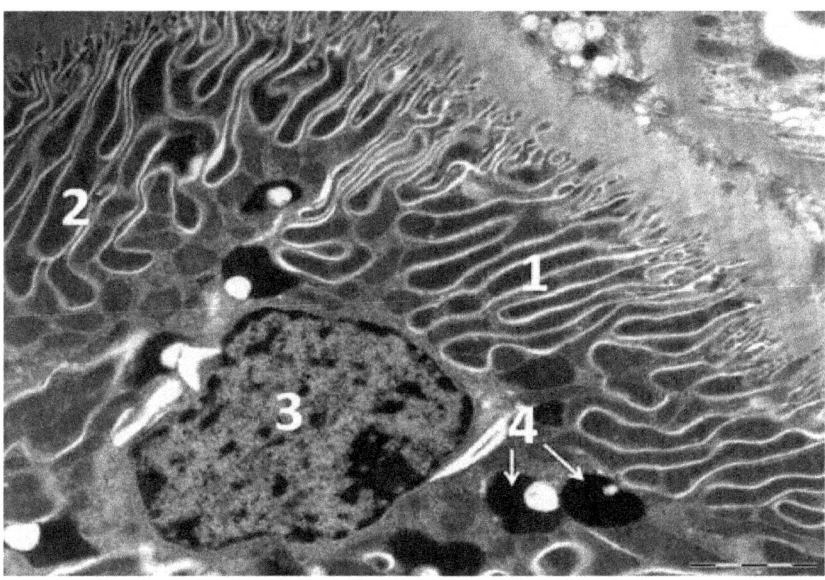

Fig. 62. Electron micrograph of the proximal tubule, control (healthy) kidney. Large euchromatic nucleus (3) with large mosaic nucleolus, 1 – basal infoldings of plasma membrane with large number of mitochondria; 2 – lateral infoldings of plasma membrane of two neighboring epithelial cell ; 4 – lysosomes in the cytoplasm. Pb Citrate +UA; orig. magn. 7100x.

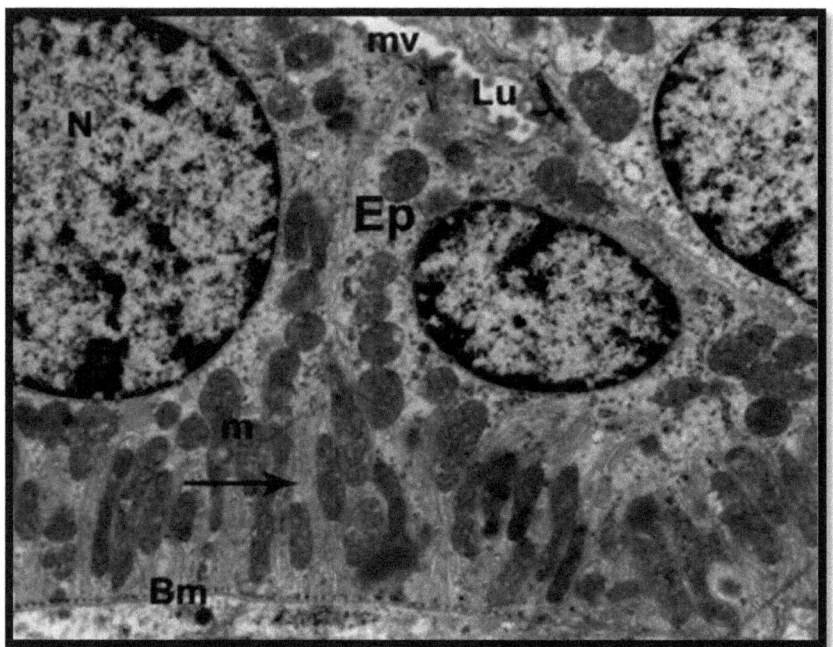

Fig. 63. An electron micrograph of a distal convoluted tubule epithelial cell (Ep) of the control kidney showing a basement membrane (Bm), short irregular microvilli (arrows), a round nucleus (N), numerous intact mitochondria (M) and lumen (Lu). (X 15000).

Ultrastructural features of the Kidney

Glomeruli

Ultrastructural examination of the renal cortex showed glomeruli with its capillary lumen a basement membrane and endothelial cell, a visceral epithelial cell with foot processes, glomeruli capsule (Glomeruli's capsule) and mesangial cell, filtration slits and intact clear urinary space .

In normal glomeruli, the visceral epithelial cells, or podocytes, have foot processes that are intact in normal glomeruli. The glomerular basement membrane (Bm) has three ultrastructural zones: the lamina densa in the middle, the lamina lucida (rara) externa, and the lamina lucida (rara) interna. The urinary space and the foot processes are at the top. Slit pore diaphragms connect the epithelial cell foot processes. The pores through the endothelial cell (En) are below the Bm. The endothelial cell nucleus sits over the origin of the mesangium .

The Proximal Convoluted Tubules

Epithelial lining cells of the proximal convoluted tubules appeared with euchromatic nuclei, tall apical microvilli and elongated mitochondria within basal enfoldings. Apical surface shows long microvilli forming a brush border towards the lumen .

The cells of the proximal convoluted tubule are cuboidal, with microvilli on their luminal side, lots of mitochondria, lateral margins very interdigitated, and an infolded membrane on their bottoms. There are canaliculi at the bases of the microvilli, with their tips pinching off to produce pinocytotic vesicles. These vesicles then fuse with lysosomes .

The Distal Convoluted Tubules

Distal convoluted tubules showed wide tubular lumen lined by epithelial cells have round euchromatic nuclei. The apical end of each distal tubule cell does not have a brush border although there may be scattered microvilli. The apical ends of distal tubule cells tend to be more distinct than those of proximal tubule cells, conferring the usual appearance of a larger, clearer lumen in each distal tubule. Distal tubule cells have a high proportion of elongated mitochondria in their cytoplasm. The plasma membranes of adjacent distal tubule cells are extensively interdigitated. As a consequence of such interdigitated cell membranes, boundaries between adjacent distal tubule cells are inconspicuous .

Contribution of Scientists

Robert Adolph Armand Tigerstedt

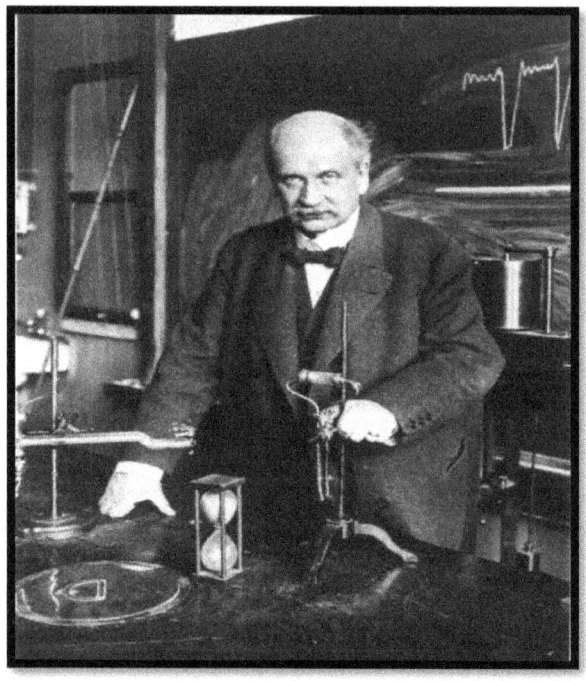

Robert Adolph Armand Tigerstedt

Born: 28 February 1853 Helsinki, Finland
Died: 12 February 1923 Helsinki, Finland
Nationality: Finnish
Alma mater: University of Helsinki
Known for: Discovery of renin

Contribution

Robert Tigerstedt, a physiologist from Finland, was the first to describe the vasopressor effects of the kidney extract he appropriately named renin in 1898. He was able to demonstrate that the injection of a kidney extract into the jugular veins of experimental rabbits resulted in a significant elevation in blood pressure. His discovery of renin went largely neglected until almost three decades later, when his results were replicated in a similar experiment using canines. Their line of renin research was interrupted for almost 40 years until the importance of the kidney in blood pressure regulation was rediscovered by Goldblatt in 1934 .

GOLDBLATT, HARRY

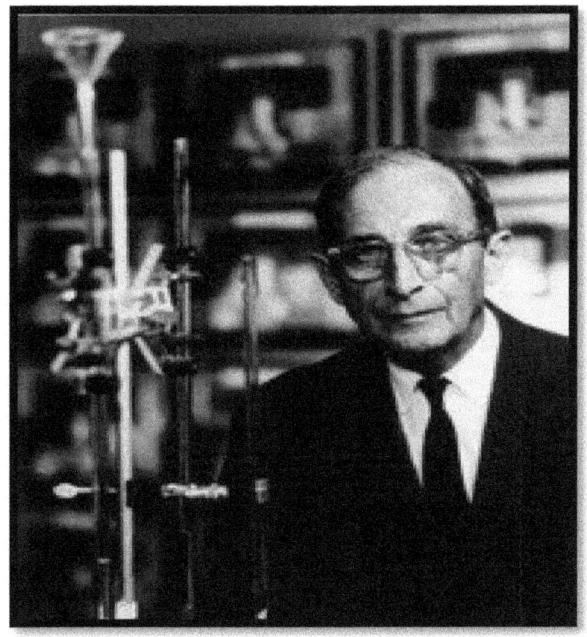

GOLDBLATT, HARRY

Harry Goldblatt

Pathologist
Born: 14 March 1891, Iowa, United States
Died: 6 January 1977
Awards: AMA Scientific Achievement Award

Main Contribution of Harry Goldblatt

Harry Goldblatt, an experimental pathologist, was best known for his work on blood pressure. In 1934, he conducted a classic experiment with the renal arteries of dogs. In the study, he constricted the renal artery with an adjustable clamp to induce an experimental hypertension that was almost identical to hypertension experienced by humans. This became known as the Goldblatt type of hypertension, and the experiment stimulated more research on the subject than almost any other medical experiment in history. From his experiment, Goldblatt concluded that variations in blood flow to the kidneys played a critical role in blood pressure elevation. This discovery allowed physicians to treat, and potentially cure, patients with hypertension, a previously unheard of premise. In 1974, the World Health

Organization established human renin (purified by Goldblatt and his associate Dr. Erwin Haas), an enzyme in the kidneys that produces a protein responsible for raising blood pressure, as the international standard for measurement, and they are now referred to as Goldblatt units.

Pancreas

Pancreas Anatomical disposition

The pancreas is an elongated, soft, flat, lobulated and yellowish gland that lies on the posterior abdominal wall, more-or-less transversely. It is a retroperitoneal structure and possesses a thin capsule. For descriptive purposes the pancreas is divided into a head, neck, body and tail. The head and tail mark the right and left extremities of the gland, respectively. The head and neck of the pancreas lie slightly to the right of the midline while the tail is to the left of the midline. The body of the pancreas passes to the left, inclining slightly upwards to become continuous with the tail. As it passes from right to left, the body of the pancreas arches across in front of the aorta and vertebral column, approximately in the transpyloric plane at the level of the first lumbar vertebra.

Microscopic structure

The pancreas is a finely lobulated gland contained within a delicate fibrous capsule. The lobules are composed of acini of serous secretory cells. The acini comprise the exocrine part of the pancreas and discharge their secretions via ductules into the principal ducts. Between the acini lie the islets of Langerhans. The islets are discrete aggregations of different secretory cell types, distinguishable by histochemical staining. The alpha cells of the islets secrete glucagon; the beta cells secrete pro-insulin (a congener of insulin). A third cell type, the delta cell, secretes somatostatin.

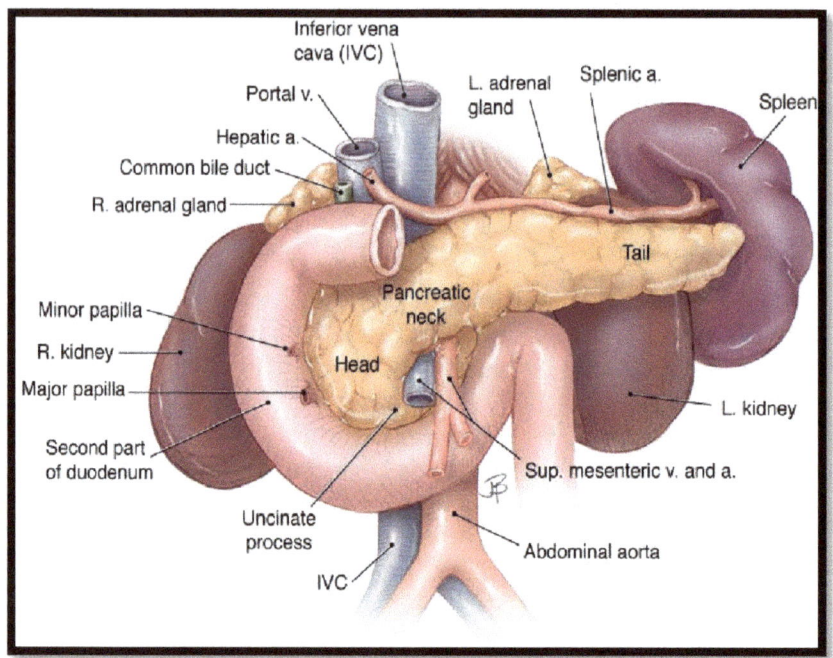

Fig. 64. Anatomic relationships of the pancreas with surrounding organs and structures Several key relationships should be noted.

Pancreas (Histological Structure)

The pancreas is an accessory organ and exocrine gland of the digestive system, as well as a hormone producing endocrine gland. It is a retroperitoneal organ consisting of five parts and an internal system of ducts. The pancreas is supplied by pancreatic arteries stemming from surrounding vessels and is innervated by the vagus nerve (CN X), celiac plexus, and superior mesenteric plexus.

Pancreas is a mixed gland formed of exocrine and endocrine parts. The exocrine part includes the pancreatic acini which secrete pancreatic enzymes; and the endocrine part includes the islets of Langerhans which secrete pancreatic hormones. Pancreatic acini consist of pyramidal cells containing basal rounded nuclei. The apical region of each pyramidal cell contains acidophilic granules (zymogenic granules), and the basal part is basophilic. The islets of Langerhans are present scattered between the acini in clusters. They are rounded or oval in configuration and appeared faintly stained with H&E. The islets are rich in blood capillaries traversing between cords of islet cells .

Pancreatic islets

Pancreatic Islets are spherical clusters of polygonal endocrine cells. On a pancreas histological slide stained with H&E, they appear as large, pale-staining cells enveloped by intensely staining, basophilic pancreatic acini. The cells of the islets are connected to each other with desmosomes and gap junctions, forming bands or cords of cells. Pancreatic islets are permeated by many fenestrated capillaries, which allow quick entry of pancreatic hormones into the blood.

There are four main types of cells in the pancreatic islets:

B (beta) cells - these cells secrete insulin and constitute about 70% of the islet cells. They are most commonly located in the central part of the islet.

A (alpha) cells - these cells secrete glucagon and constitute 15-20% of the islet cells. They are usually larger than B cells and most commonly located peripherally in the islet.

D (delta) cells - these cells secrete somatostatin and constitute 5-10% of the islet cells. They are located diffusely throughout the islet but most commonly in the periphery.

PP (pancreatic polypeptide) cells - these cells secrete pancreatic polypeptide and constitute <5% of the islet cells. They are mostly located within the head of the pancreas.

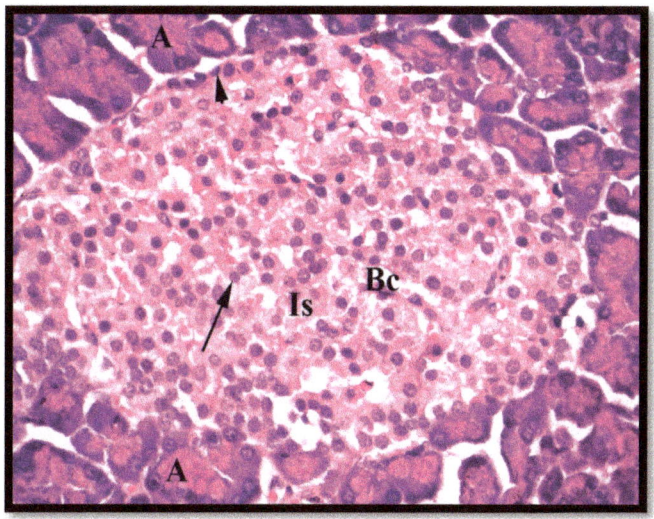

Fig. 65. A photomicrograph of pancreas from control rat (I) showing an islet of Langerhans (Is) which appears as pale stained rounded area surrounded by darkly

stained pancreatic acini (A). The islet of langerhans consists of cords of cells separated by blood capillaries (Bc). The β-cells (arrow) are located mainly in the central zone of the islet with rounded and lighter nuclei. The α-cells (arrow head) are located peripherally with oval darkly stained nuclei (H & E stain X 400)

Ultrastructure of Pancreatic Acinar cells

Ultrastructure of control pancreas showed acinar cells with euchromatic nuclei, well-developed cisternae of rough endoplasmic reticulum, mitochondria and numerous electron dense secretory granules of variable sizes in the apical part.

The pancreatic islets of Langerhans of control rats showed that beta cells are mainly distributed at the central parts of the islets and represent the majority of the islet cells. The cytoplasm embodies numerous specific membrane-bound granules, which contain insulin hormone. The core of granules is electron-dense, and a wide clear space (electron-lucent area) is seen between the core and the bounding membrane of granules. Golgi apparatus, rER, mitochondria with condensed matrix, lysosomes and other cytoplasmic components appeared normal in the beta-cells of control rat's pancreas. They have rounded large and light peripherally located nuclei.

The alpha cells contain dense round granules that contained glucagon hormone. The granule contents consist of round electron dense core that is closely surrounded by the peripherally granule limiting membrane. The cells have oval or indented nuclei.

The somatostatin or delta cells (δ) are polygonal in shape with eccentric nuclei. The δ cells are smaller in size than both α and β cells. They have rounded small electron dense granules.

The polypeptide cells (PP) are the last type of islet cells which are characterized by small spherical granules and exhibit a homogenous electron dense material. They have small rounded nuclei.

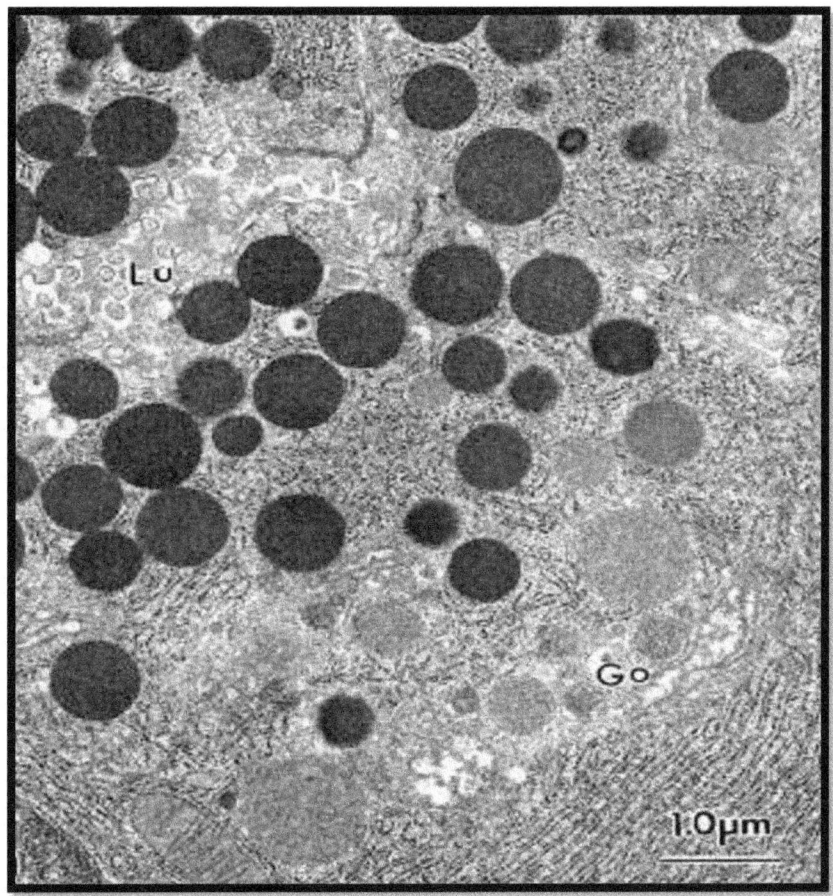

Fig. 66. Electron microscopy of exocrine pancreatic tissue of normal rats. Golgi is well developed, granules are normal, and acinar lumen contains secretory material as well as many microvilli (1 1 9 0 0 X). Lu., lumen ; Gol., Golgi.

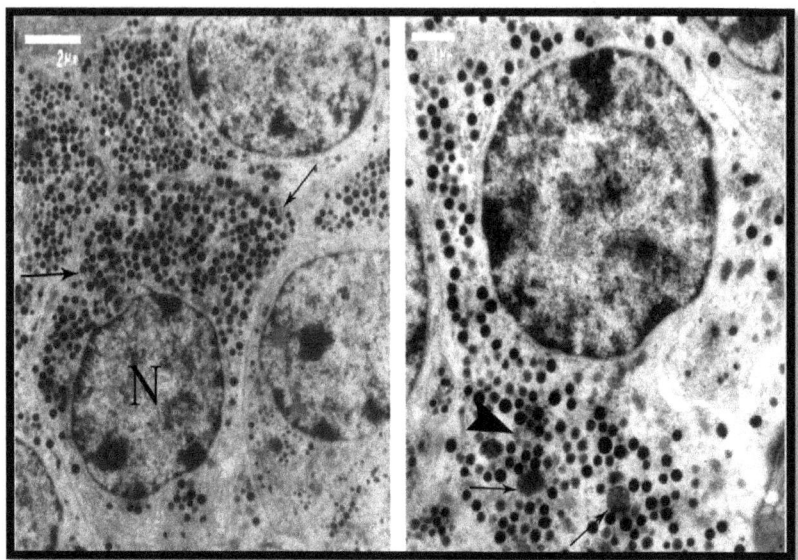

Fig. 67. Alpha cells. Electron micrograph of rat pancreas showing (a) the cytoplasm of control a cells with numerous secretory granules (arrows) of electron dense core and surrounded by narrow halo. Notice the round euchromatic nucleus (N). Scale bar= 2 μm. (b) Mitochondria (arrows) of control a cells and numerous secretory granules (arrow head). Scale bar = 1 μm.

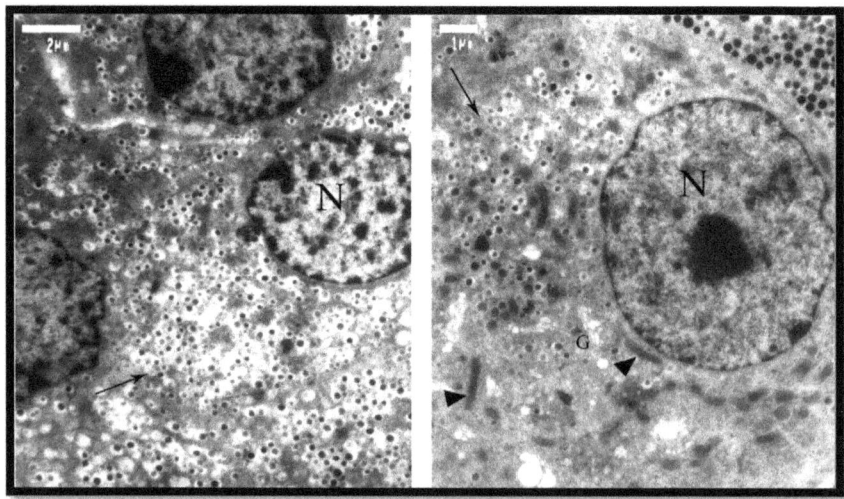

Fig. 68. Beta cells. Electron micrograph of rat pancreas showing (a and b) control Islets of Langerhans were formed mainly of b-cells. Their cytoplasm contains numerous electron dense secretory granules surrounded by wide lucent halo (arrow), mitochondria (arrow head), Golgi apparatus (G) and euchromatic nucleus (N). scale bar = 2 & 1 μm   respectively.

Contribution of Scientists
derick Grant Banting

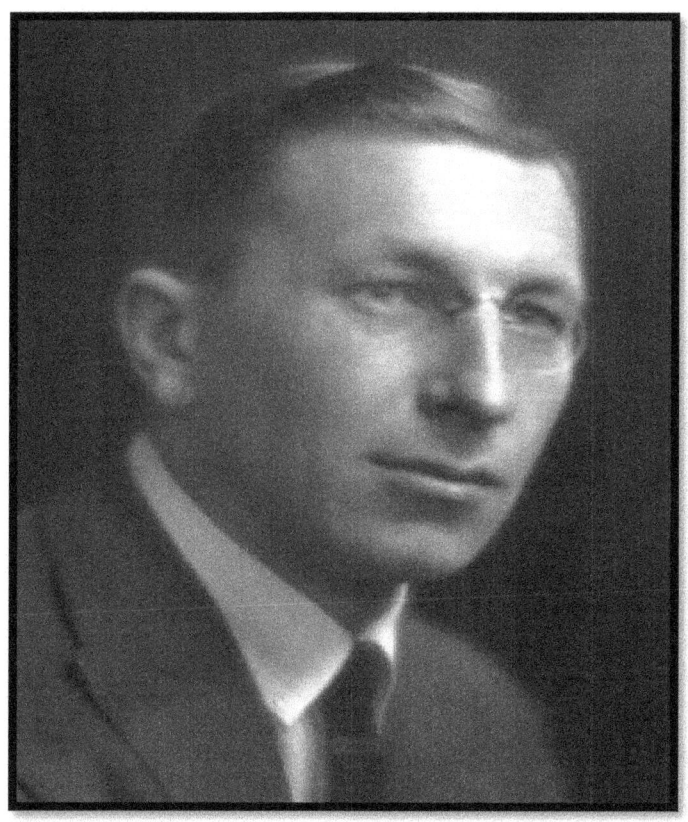

derick Grant Banting
The Nobel Prize in Physiology or Medicine 1923
Born: 14 November 1891, Alliston, Canada
Died: 21 February 1941, Newfoundland, Canada
Affiliation at the time of the award: University of Toronto, Toronto, Canada

John James Rickard Macleod

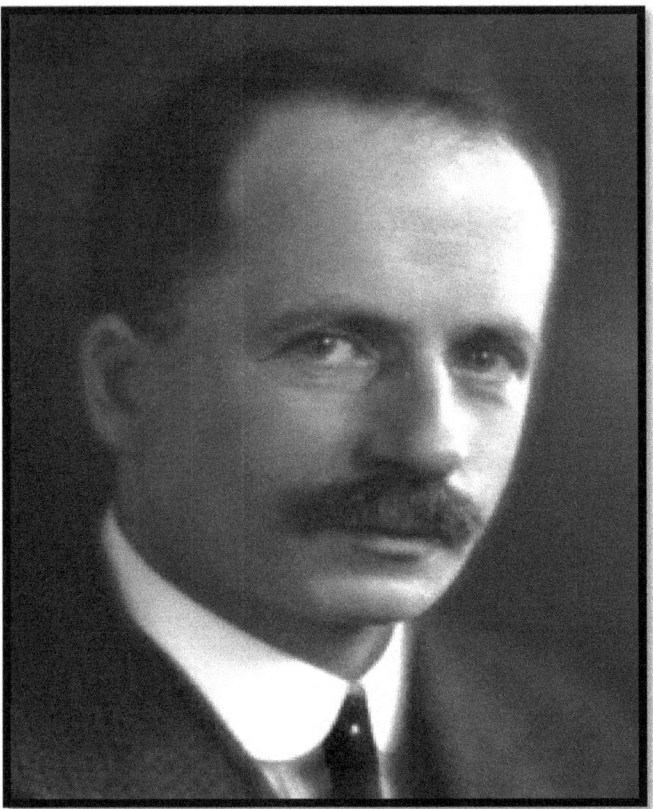

John James Rickard Macleod
The Nobel Prize in Physiology or Medicine 1923
Born: 6 September 1876, Cluny, Scotland
Died: 16 March 1935, Aberdeen, Scotland
Affiliation at the time of the award: University of Toronto, Toronto, Canada

IMPORTANT CONTRIBUTION OF THE SCIENTISTS

Insulin was the first peptide hormone discovered. Frederick Banting and Charles Herbert Best, working in the laboratory of J. J. R. Macleod at the University of Toronto, were the first to isolate insulin from dog pancreas in 1921. Frederick Sanger sequenced the amino acid structure in 1951, which made insulin the first protein to be fully sequenced. The crystal structure of insulin in the solid state was determined by Dorothy Hodgkin in 1969. Insulin is also the first protein to be chemically synthesised and produced by DNA recombinant technology. It is on the WHO Model List of Essential Medicines, the most important medications needed in a basic health system.

LIVER

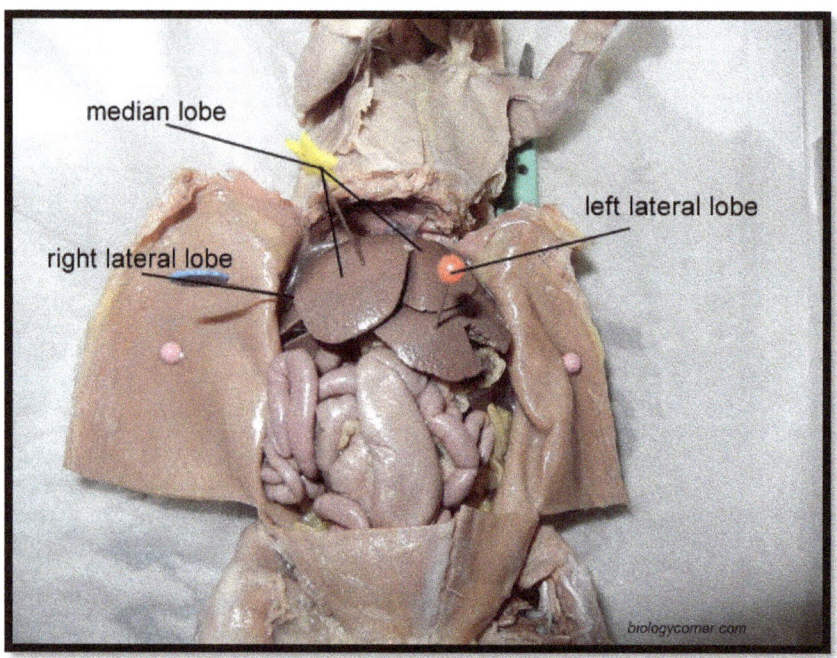

Fig. 69. Anatomical Position of Liver lobes within the abdominal cavity of rat.

Anatomy of Liver

Liver is a solid dark reddish-brown half-moon shaped organ. It contains two lobes i.e. right and left lobe which is separated by the falciform ligament.

Each lobe is further divided into many lobules which flows into the hepatic duct and has millions of hepatocytes.

The outer layer of the liver is covered by fibrous tissue called Glisson's capsule which protects the liver from physical damage (Glisson's capsule is in turn covered by peritoneum).

Liver receives blood by means of two ways i.e. hepatic artery and portal vein.

- **Hepatic Artery** – It carries oxygen-rich blood from the heart to liver.

- **Portal Vein** – It carries nutrient-rich blood from the digestive system to the liver.

Gall bladder is present under the liver. The bile produced by the liver is carried by bile ducts towards the hepatic duct. It joins with the cystic duct from the gall bladder and forms common bile duct which opens into the small intestine.

Most of the bile produced by the liver is stored in the gall bladder by peristalsis.

HISTOLOGICAL STRUCTURES

The liver is the largest organ of the body, constituting 2-5% of the adult body weight.

It is surrounded by connective tissue, designated as Glisson's capsule. It is composed of polygonal lobules separated by connective tissue. At the periphery of the lobule, are regions that consist of bile ducts, lymphatics, nerves and branches of the hepatic artery and the portal vein. At the center of the lobule is the central vein. Hepatocytes (parenchymal cells) are the basic structural component of the liver, representing 60% of the total cell number and 80% of the total liver volume. They are arranged radially within the lobule to form cellular plates, between which the liver capillaries and the sinusoids are located.

Microscopically, each liver lobe is seen to be made up of hepatic lobules. The lobules are roughly hexagonal, and consist of plates of hepatocytes, and sinusoids radiating from a central vein towards an imaginary perimeter of interlobular portal triads. The central vein joins to the hepatic vein to carry blood out from the liver. A distinctive component of a lobule is the portal triad, which can be found running along each of the lobule's corners. The portal triad, consists of the hepatic artery, the portal vein, and the common bile duct.

Histology, the study of microscopic anatomy, shows two major types of liver cell: parenchymal cells and nonparenchymal cells. About 70–85% of the liver volume is occupied by parenchymal hepatocytes. Nonparenchymal cells constitute 40% of the total number of liver cells but only 6.5% of its volume. The liver sinusoids are lined with two types of cell, sinusoidal endothelial cells, and phagocytic Kupffer cells. The sinusoidal cells are the predominant non-parenchymal cells, comprising about 35% of the total cell number and about 17% of the total volume of the liver. These cells are divided into sinusoidal endothelial cells (44%), Kupffer cells (33%), stellate cells (10-25%) and hepatic NK cells (5%).

Additionally, intrahepatic lymphocytes are often present in the sinusoidal lumen.

Functions of Liver

Liver is an organ as well as gland which performs multiple functions i.e. as an organ it performs chemical actions required for the body and as a gland, it secretes chemicals required for the body.

- Liver along with pharynx and intestine helps to digest, absorb and process the food.
- Bile secreted by the liver helps in fat metabolism, production of cholesterol and triglycerides.
- Iron is stored in the liver/bone marrow to make red blood cells.
- Bile helps to absorb vitamin K which helps in clotting of blood.
- Liver stores vitamin A, D, K and B12.
- Insulin is produced by the pancreas which helps to maintain glucose level.
- Liver can regenerate its organ after an injury or surgery.
- Filters toxic chemicals and bacteria from the body.

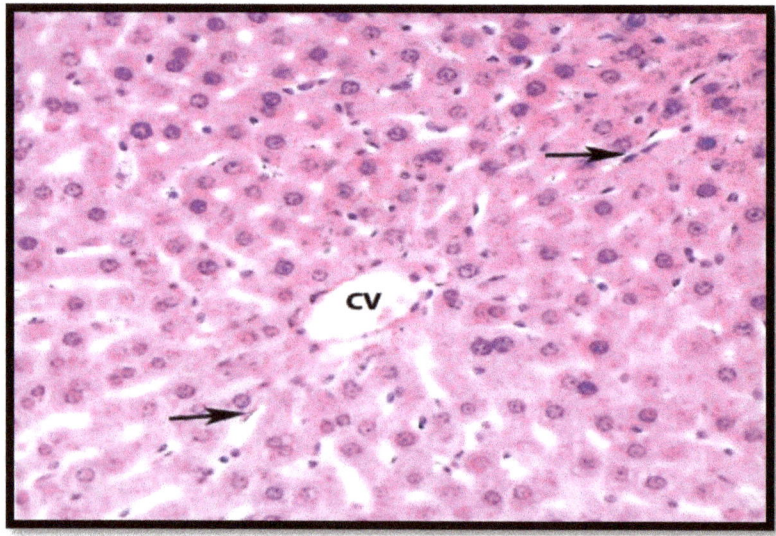

Fig. 70. Liver section showing normal polyhedral hepatocytes and their radiation from the central vein (CV) with eosinophilic cytoplasm and centrally located nuclei. Between the cords of hepatocytes, blood sinusoids are often seen with phagocytic Kuffer cells (arrows) (H&E, X400).

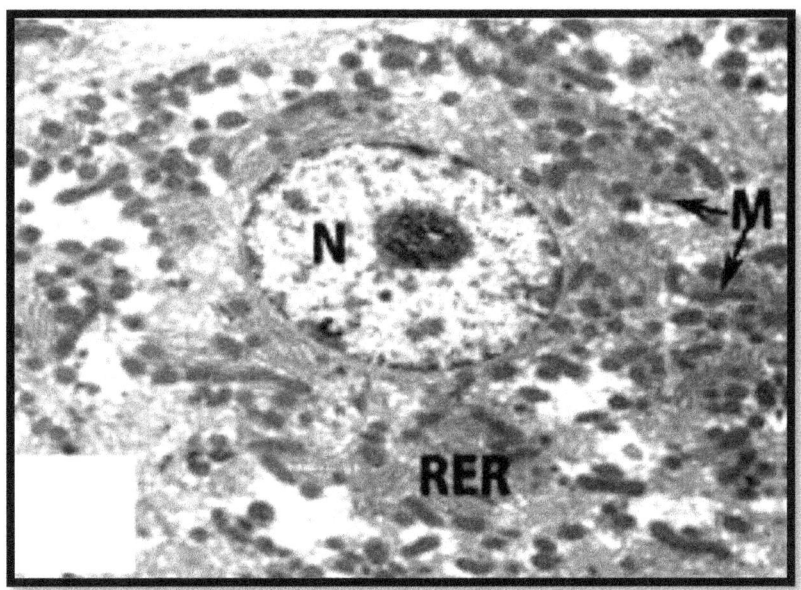

Fig. 71. Ultrastructure . Control rat showing; centrally located rounded nuclei (N), normal distribution of hetero and euchromatin and well-developed RER and mitochondria with dense matrices and vary in shape (X3600).

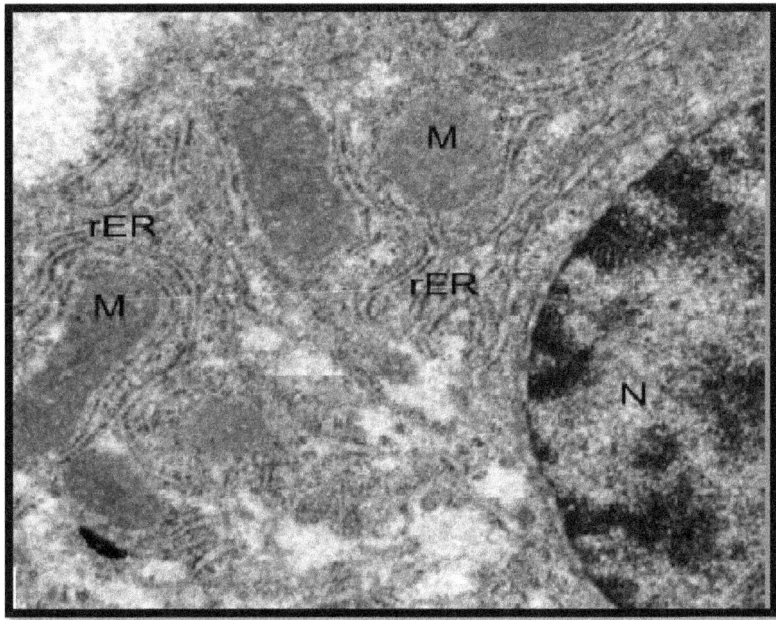

Fig. 72. Electron micrograph of liver rat from control group showing part of the hepatocyte with nucleus (N), parallel cisternae of rough endoplasmic reticulum (rER) and numerous mitochondria (M). x7500

Kupffer cells :

- triangular or star shaped, smaller, migrating cells in the sinusoids
- are part of the immune system – diffuse mononuclear phagocyte system (MPS)
- uptake and degrade foreign and potentially harmful substances
- proliferate and enlarge in response to hepatocyte damage, bacterial toxins, etc.
- uptake senescent red blood cells and break down hemoglobin

Ultrastructure of Hepatocyte

Electron micrographs of liver from control animals revealed characteristic normal hepatocyte ultrastructure. The hepatocytes contain a rather centrally located rounded or oval nucleus with normal distribution of hetero- and euchromatin. The nucleus is surrounded by parallel cisternae of rough endoplasmic reticulum (rER) which is arranged in parallel stacks. . The mitochondria were found in close association with the rER, varying from circular to elongated form. Some lipid droplets were present in the cytoplasm which was mainly filled with glycogen.

The cytoplasm is acidophilic in routine H&E staining, dotted with basophilic regions represented by rough endoplasmic reticulum (rER) and ribosomes. In addition, hepatocytes contain the following organelles:

Smooth endoplasmic reticulum (sER), which is essential in toxin degradation and conjugation, as well as cholesterol synthesis.

Mitochondria (up to 1000/cell)

Golgi network, which is composed of approximately 50 small Golgi units. They contain granules with very low density lipoprotein and bile precursors.

Peroxisomes, which contain oxidases and catalases. These enzymes are responsible for detoxification reactions taking place in the liver, for example, that of alcohol.

Glycogen deposits, which are lost in during H&E preparations, leaving irregular stained areas.

Lipid droplets

Lysosomes, which are responsible for iron storage under the form of ferritin.

Contribution of Scientists

Karl Wilhem von Kupffer

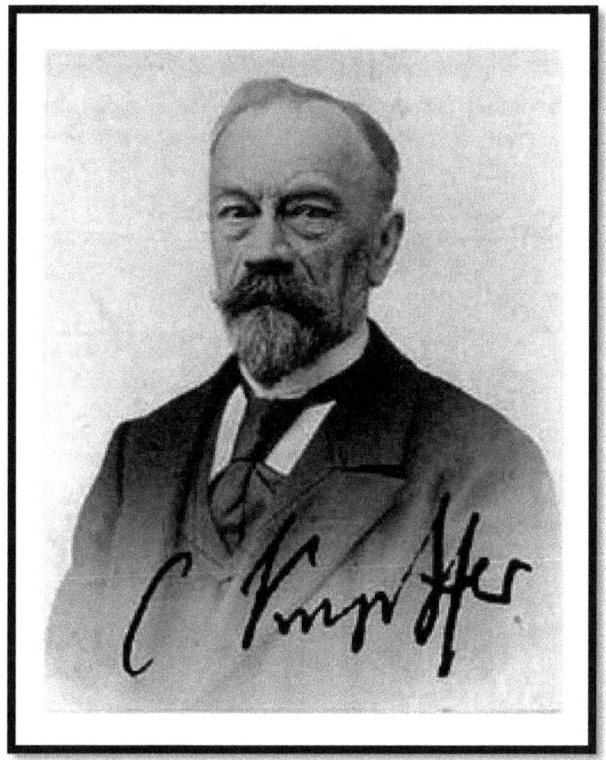

Karl Wilhem von Kupffer (Germany)

Born : on November 14, 1829,
Died : on 16th of December in 1902 at the age of 73,
Fields : physiology and anatomy

Discovery:

In regards to his discovery of "Kupffer cells" in 1876, he initially suggested that this type of cell belonged to a group of perivascular cells (pericytes) of the connective tissues or to the adventitial cells. Shortly afterwards, pathologist Tadeusz Browicz (1847-1928) from Jagellonian University in Krakow, correctly identified them as macrophages.

Kupffer cells, the resident macrophage in the liver, comprise the largest population of resident tissue macrophages in the body. First described by Karl Wilhelm von Kupffer in 1876 as "sternzellen" (star cells or stellate cells), Kupffer cells were first thought to be a part of the endothelium of the liver blood vessels. It was not until 1898 that Tadeusz Browiecz correctly identified them as macrophages. Kupffer cells play a critical role in the innate immune response; their localization in the hepatic sinusoid allows them to efficiently phagocytize pathogens entering from the portal or arterial circulation. Kupffer cells also serve as a first line of defence against particulates and immunoreactive material passing from the gastrointestinal tract via the portal circulation and may be considered as a final component in gut barrier function. Kupffer cells thus play a major anti-inflammatory role by preventing the movement of these gut-derived immunoreactive substances from travelling past the hepatic sinusoid.

Pineal Gland

The Pineal gland

The pineal gland is a small endocrine gland located within the brain. Its main secretion is melatonin, which regulates the circadian rhythm of the body. It is also thought to produce hormones that inhibit the action of other endocrine glands in the body.

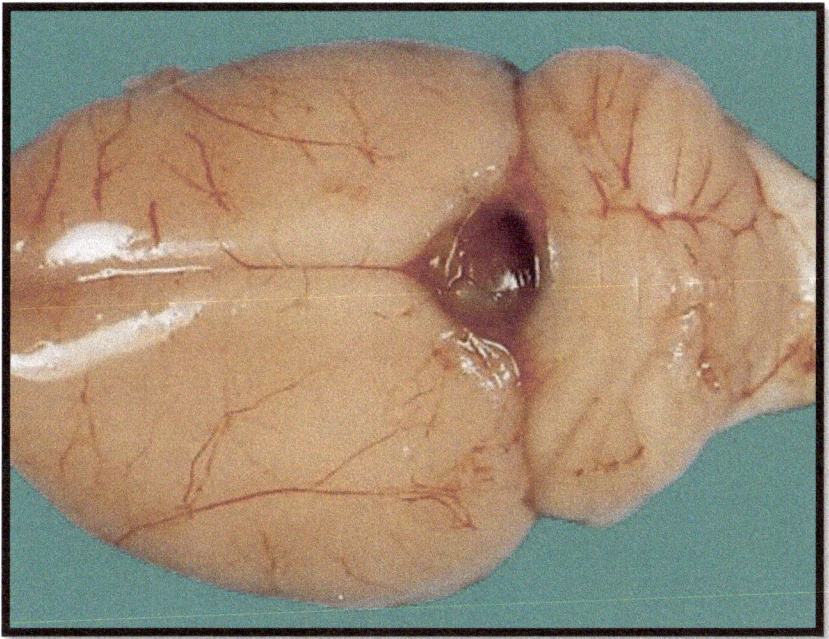

Fig. Anatomical position of the pineal gland of rat from dissection

Anatomy

The epiphysis cerebri or pineal gland is a reddish-grey, approximately 5 – 8 mm long, pine cone-like structure that is located in the diencephalic part of the prosencephalon (forebrain). The gland was formed as an outward growth of the roof of the third ventricle. Therefore, the gland rests between the posterior aspects of the thalami as it projects posteriorly from the wall of the third ventricle.

Histology

The pineal gland is encased by pia mater and lobulated by its connective tissue septae that projects into the gland. Within the epiphysis cerebri, there are pinealocytes and neuroglia cells. The pinealocytes account for approximately 95% of the cellular content of the gland. They are irregularly shaped with peripheral processes, and lightly staining large round nuclei. Pinealocytes are primarily concerned with the photo-regulated production of melatonin. This hormone works with the body's circadian rhythm (which is controlled by the suprachiasmatic nucleus of the hypothalamus) to regulate the cycle of sleep and wakefulness. Additionally, some researchers believe that melatonin may alter sexual development in humans, contribute to thermoregulation, and cellular metabolism.

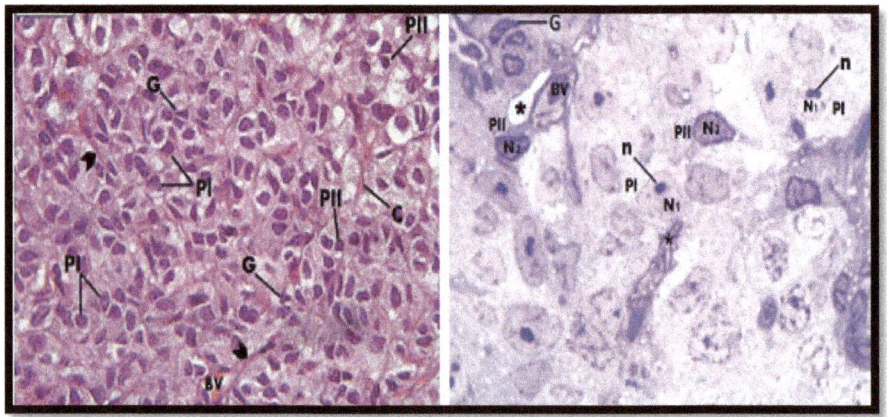

Fig. 73 A and B. Photomicrographs of pineal gland from GI showing:

A. plates of closely packed pinealocytes. Pinealocytes type I (PI) and pinealocytes type II (PII) appear within parenchymal lobules (circle), separated by fibrous septae (arrowheads) containing blood vessels (BV). Glial cells (G) scattered among pinealocytes whereas the blood capillaries (C) are situated among parenchymal cells. (H & E : x 400)

B. tightly packed pinealocytes within the parenchymal lobules in semithin section. Pinealocytes type I (PI); pale cytoplasm surrounding large euchromatic nuclei (N1) with prominent nucleoli (n). Pinealocytes type II (PII) demonstrate darkly-stained nuclei (N2) and appear near the perivascular space (*) which surrounds the blood vessels (BV) seen between the parenchymal lobules. Glial cells (G), deeply-stained nuclei. (Toluidine blue : x 1000)

Secretion of Pineal Gland:

The pineal gland secretes a single hormone—melatonin (not to be confused with the pigment melanin). This simple hormone is special because its secretion is dictated by light. Researchers have determined that melatonin has two primary functions in humans—to help control your circadian (or biological) rhythm and regulate certain reproductive hormones.

Ultrastructure of the rat pineal gland

The nucleus of Type I pinealocytes displayed numerous infoldings in its envelope. Mitochondria varying greatly in size and shape occupied a large part of the cytoplasm. Granular endoplasmic reticulum formed short cisterns, either isolated or in stacks. Cells in young adult glands frequently displayed large clusters of smooth endoplasmic reticulum located in the periphery near the cell membrane . The Golgi complex occupied a large area near the nucleus. No centrioles or cilia were found in adult rats. Dense bodies or lysosomes within the Type I pinealocyte obviously increased in number with age . Lipid droplets whose size and density differed from one cell to another were also found in the cytoplasm of this cell type . Larger lipid droplets were found in older animals.

Type II pinealocytes were characterised by their great nuclear and cytoplasmic density as well as by their cytoplasmic processes. Contact surfaces between two cell bodies or between a cell body and a process showed gap-like junctions. The nucleus of the Type II pinealocyte was genelally ovoid . Infoldings in the nuclear envelope, sometimes deep and complex, were frequently found in older rats. The nucleolus was very small and generally peripherally placed. The dense cytoplasm displayed cisterns of granular endoplasmic reticulum containing flocculent material and were very rich in ribosomes. In younger rats, there were a few dense bodies in the cytoplasm of the soma. With increasing age, small lipofuscin granules appeared . Centrioles and even cilia were relatively frequent in Type II pinealocytes. Some large round lipid droplets were also observed, mostly in younger adults. Vacuoles surrounded by a double membrane characteristic of this cell type were also found. Filaments were sometimes observed, mostly in the processes.

Calvo, J. And Boya, J. (1984) . Ultrastructure of the pineal gland in the adult rat J.Anat. ; 138(3) : 405-409

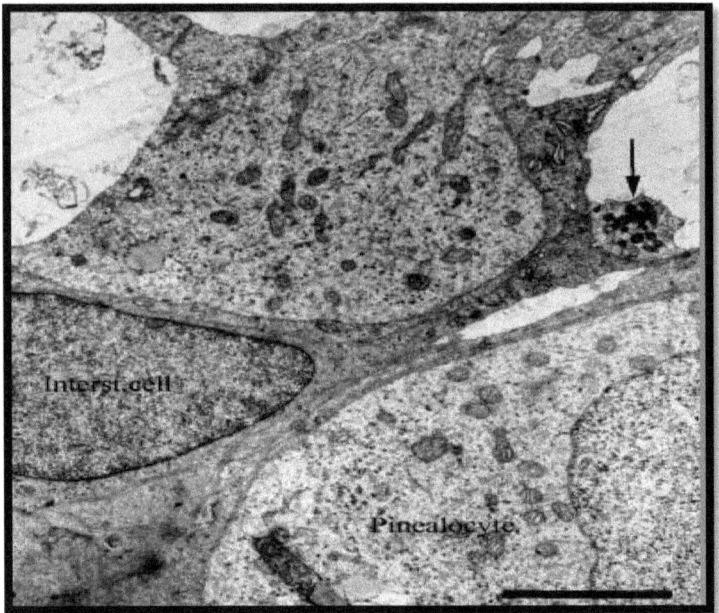

Fig. 74. Electron micrograph of the rat pineal gland showing an interstitial cell (*Interst. cell*) located between pinealocytes with more electron-lucent cytoplasm. A club-shaped terminal of a pinealocyte process is seen (*arrow*). Scale bar 5 μm

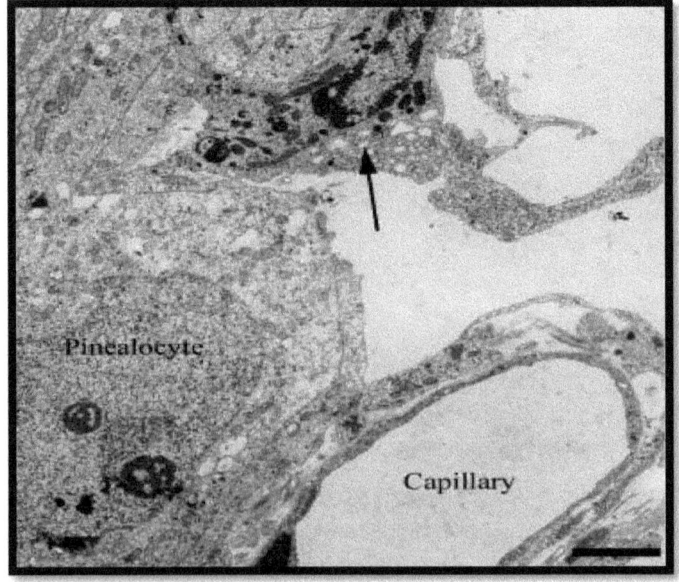

Fig. 75. Electron micrograph of the rat pineal gland showing a perivascularly located phagocyte (*arrow*). Note the high number of dense bodies in the cytoplasm. *Scale bar* 3.5 μm

PITUITARY GLAND

Anatomical position of the pituitary gland

The pituitary gland (the hypophysis) is a major gland of the endocrine system. It secretes hormones that control the actions of other endocrine organs and various tissues around the body.

The pituitary gland of the rat is located in the midline at the base of the brain on the sella turcica, which is rather flat in this animal. Superiorly, it is connected with the hypothalamus by the stalk. The pituitary gland of the rat is divided into three major anatomical parts: the pars distalis, the pars intermedia, and the pars nervosa. The pars tuberalis, composed of cells resembling those of the pars distalis, is present around the stalk up to the hypothalamus.

The vasculature of the pituitary gland is complex and unique. Whilst the anterior lobe and posterior lobe have the same venous drainage (anterior and posterior hypophyseal veins), they have an individual arterial supply:

The infundibulum and posterior pituitary gland receive a rich blood supply from many arteries. Of these, the major vessels are the superior hypophyseal artery, infundibular artery and inferior hypophyseal artery.

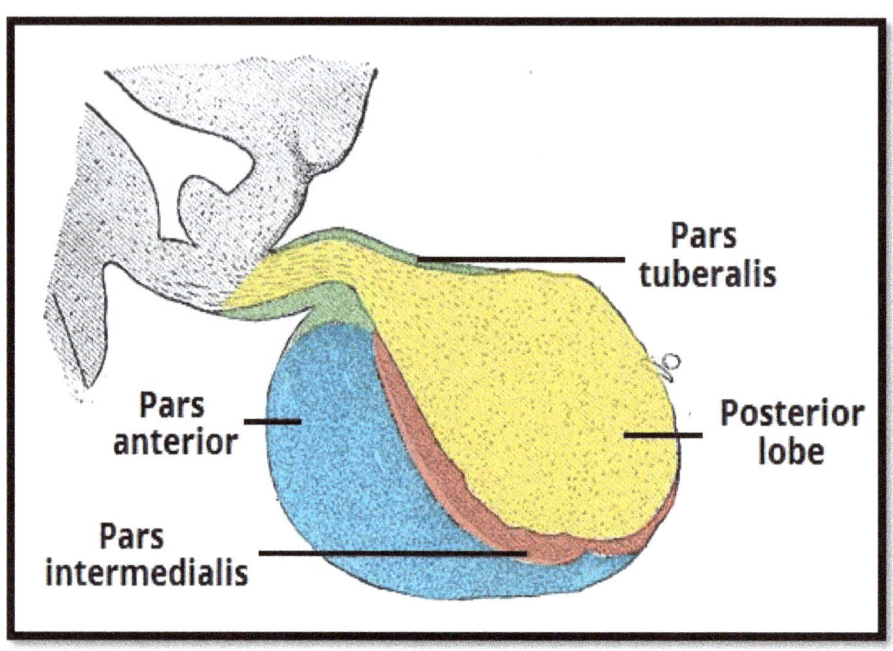

Fig. 76. The structure of the pituitary gland (Diagrammatic).

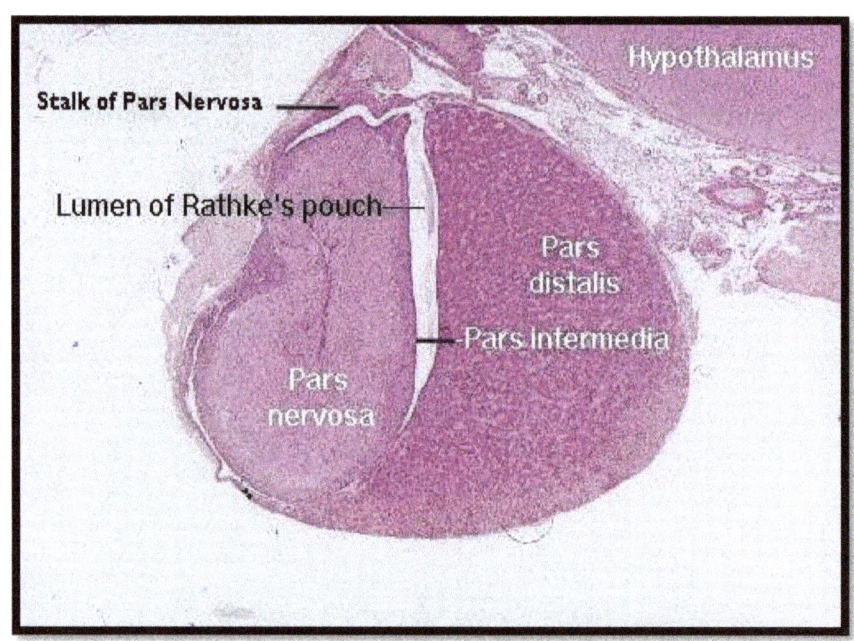

Fig. 77. Anatomical structure of the Pituitary gland

Histological structures of the adenohypophyses

Adenohypophysis (Pars Anterior, Anterior Lobe)

The pituitary gland in adults has a distinct histological appearance, reflecting its divergent origin. The adenohypophysis (pars anterior, anterior lobe) is characterised by well-demarcated acini that usually contain a mixture of different hormone-producing cells. This nested pattern is best appreciated in reticulin preparations, which delineate the borders of the acini. The cellular heterogeneity within acini may be demonstrated histochemically in PAS-OG or preparations which were widely used before the adoption of antibody-based stains. Corticotroph cells are generally strongly basophilic (PAS-positive), somatotroph and lactotroph cells mostly acidophilic (orangeophilic), whilst gonadotrophs and thyrotrophs may be basophilic or chromophobe (reacting with neither acid nor basic stains). There is no perfect match of hormone-expression and type or degree of chromophilia; some chromophobe cells may represent degranulated chromophil cells or precursor cells. In a normal adult adenohypophysis approximately 10% of endocrine cells are basophils, 40% acidophils and 50% chromophobes. Although most acini contain a mixture of different hormone-producing cells, there is evidence of zonation. The lateral wings of the gland mostly contain somatotrophs and lactotrophs, whilst corticotrophs are concentrated in the median mucoid wedge, which at its anterior border (the rostral tip) harbours clusters of thyrotrophs. Gonadotroph (LH/FSH) cells are diffusely scattered throughout the gland.

CELL TYPES OF THE ANTERIOR PITUITARY GLAND

Acidophils	Cells that contain the polypeptide hormones:
	Somatotropes which produce growth hormone
	Lactotropes which produce prolactin
Basophils	Cells that contain the glycoprotein hormones:
	Thyrotropes which produce thyroid stimulating hormone
	Gonadotropes which produce luteinizing hormone or follicle-stimulating hormone
	Corticotropes which produce adrenocorticotrophic hormone
	Due the high carbohydrate content of the hormones

within acidophils, they also stain bright purple with PAS stains.

Chromophobes — These are cells that have minimal or no hormonal content. Many of the chromophobes may be acidophils or basophils that have degranulated and thereby are depleted of hormone. Some chromophobes may also represent stem cells that have not yet differentiated into hormone-producing cells.

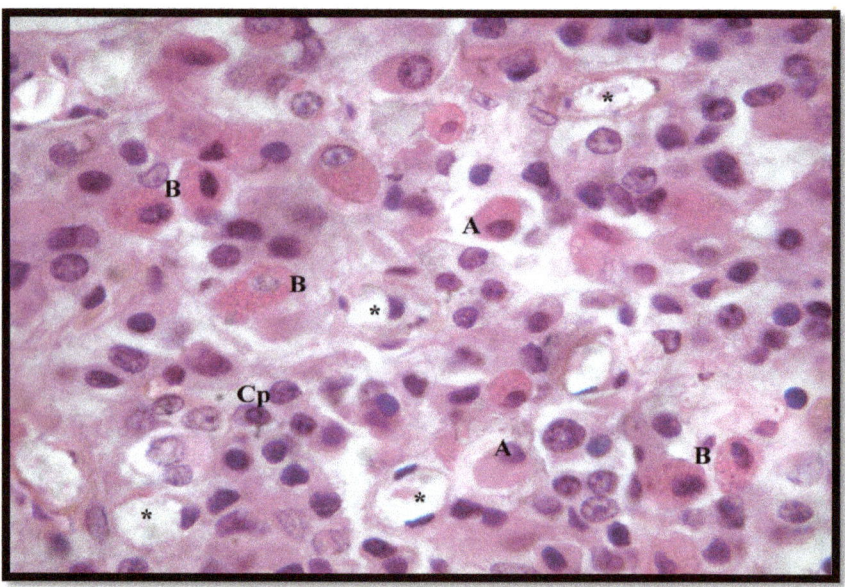

Fig. 78. A photomicrograph of a section in the control adult rat pars distalis of pituitary gland showing clusters of two main populations of cells; those with strongly staining cytoplasm {chromophils; acidophils (A) with acidophilic cytoplasm and eccentric nuclei and basophils basophilic granular cytoplasm and eccentric nuclei (B)} and those with weakly staining cytoplasm (chromophobes Cp). Notice the blood sinusoids (*). (H&E X1000).

Ultrastructure of the Pituitary cell types

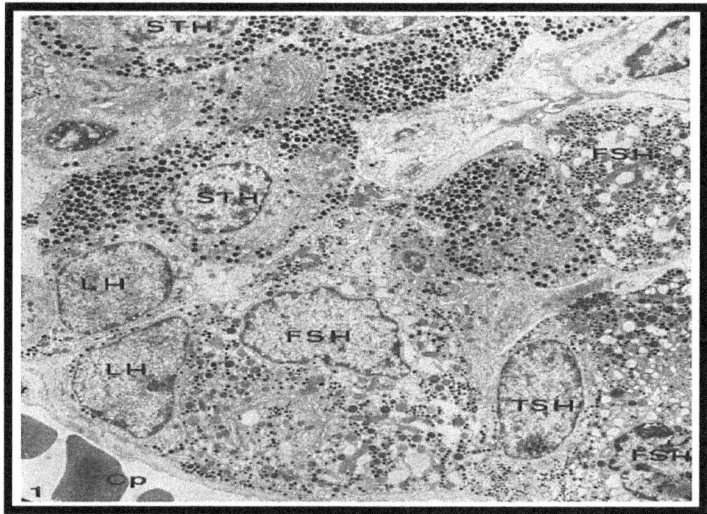

Fig. 79. Low power electron micrograph of an anterior pituitary gland STH somatotrophs; FSH follicle-stimulating gonadotroph; LH luteinizing gonadotroph; TSH thyrotroph

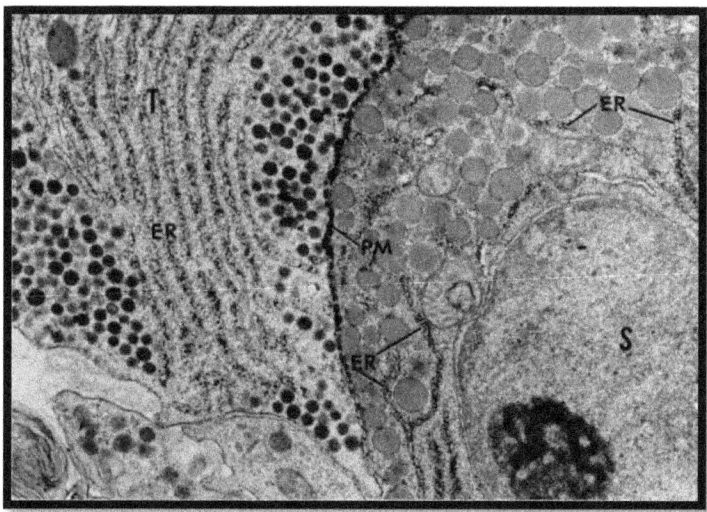

Fig. 80. Portions of a thyrotroph (T) and somatotroph (S) occupy most of the field. The parallel ar- rays of ER in thyrotrophs and ER of somatotroph show NDP ase reaction product (ER). Note the contrast in size of secretory granules of the two cell types. Reaction product is at plasma membranes and the interspace between the two cells (PM). X20,000.

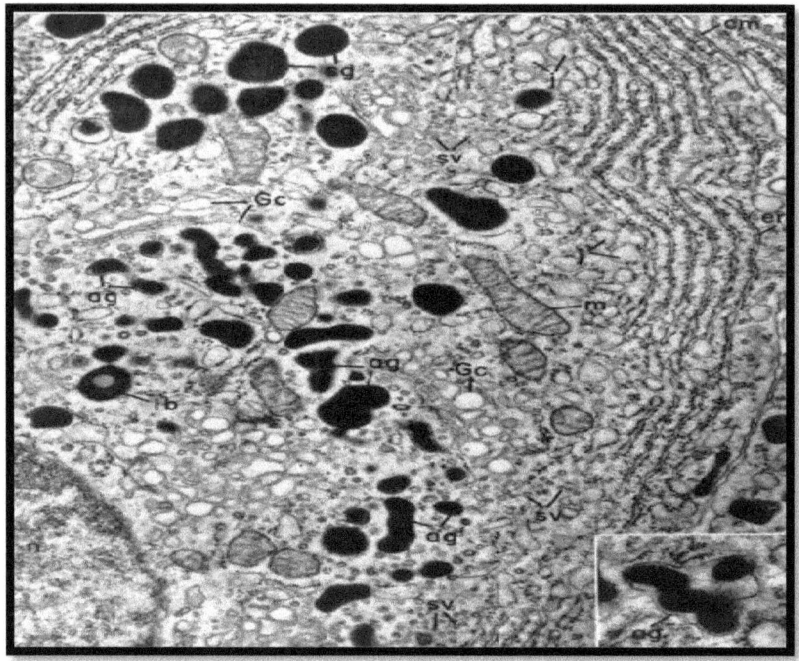

Fig. 81. Mammotroph cell from the anterior pituitary gland of a lactating rat. This micrograph illustrates the morphological complexity of the regulated secretory pathway, and the diVerent types of ISGs. ER endoplasmic reticulum; CM cell membrane; SG secretory granule; SV smooth vesicles; VE vesicle; LB lytic body. Reproduced from the J Cell Biol., 1966, 31:319–347.

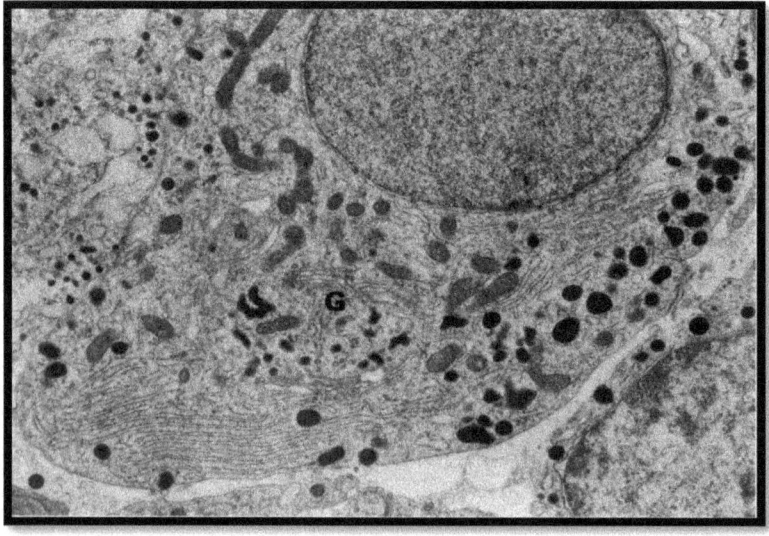

Fig. 82. A prolactin cell from a control rat. G, Golgi region. x IO 300.

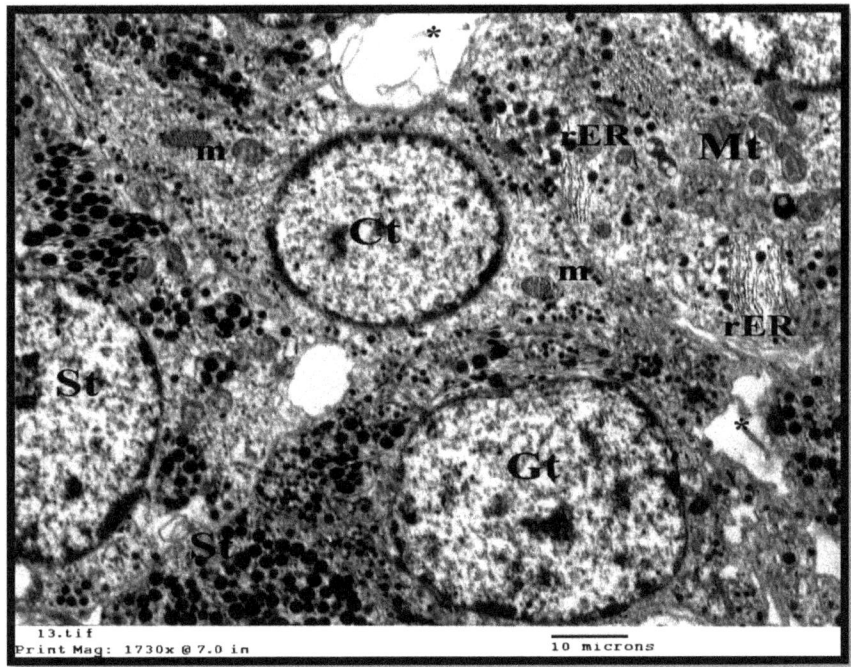

Fig. 83. An electron micrograph of an ultrathin section in the control adult rat pars distalis of pituitary gland showing an elongated corticotroph (Ct) with central nucleus, dense oval mitochondria (m) and small sparse dense uniform secretory granules located at the extreme periphery, a mammotroph (Mt) with scattered rER, mitochondria and secretory granules pleomorphic in size and shape. Notice the blood sinusoid (*), somatotrophs (St), gonadotroph (Gt) with their characteristic features. (X2000)

Rat adenohypophyseal cell types (ultrastructural features)

Lactotrophs

Typical lactotroph with immature secretory granules associated with the trans face of Golgi stacks with numerous polymorphic mature secretory granules (500-900 nm) being stored in the cytoplasm. Irregular shaped secretory granules surrounded by Golgi saccules are immunolabeled with colloidal gold particles.

Somatotrophs

Ultrastructural examination of somatotroph cells showed that these cells were similar in each group Based on the size of the secretion granules, two types of somatotroph cells could be seen: A : cells with large secretory granules (diameter, 250-350 nm) and cells with large and small secretory granules (diameter, 250-350 and 100-150 nm) and B: Somatotroph cell with abundant round secretory granules ranging from 200 to 350 nm in diameter. In both cases, cells were round or oval in shape, with rounded nuclei. GH cells with larger secretion granules were densely granulated, while somatotroph cells with smaller secretion granules were sparsely granulated. Somatotroph containing numerous spherical secretory granules immunolabeled with growth hormone antiserum.

(Reproduced from Bonaterra et al., 1998; with permission from Exp Clin Endocrinol Diabetes).

Corticotrophs

In the control animals of both sexes cells with the characteristic appearance of Siperstein corticotrophs were easily identified. These were stellate with processes surrounding other cells. The secretory granules were often arranged in a single row along the cell membrane. The most striking features of the corticotrophs lie in the characters of secretory granules. The granules measuring 150-250 mµ in dimension are distributed thoroughly in the cytoplasm and exhibit various electron densities. Rough endoplasmic reticulum was lamellar. Mitochondria were slender and often of irregular shape. No obvious differences were identified between male and female rats.

Thyrotrophs

The thyrotrophs had a polyhedral outline and small spherical secretory granules (100-150 nm in diameter) that have been proven to contain TSH immunologically. Intracytoplasmic secretory granules were located along the cell surface and were relatively few in number as compared to the other anterior pituitary cells. However, they were often arranged in two or more rows, and unevenly distributed.

Gonadotrophs

Only one type of gonadotroph could be identified, by electron microscopy, in the anterior pituitary of control rats. Gonadotrophs were the largest cell type in the adenohypophysis. Most gonadotrophs were located adjacent to capillaries. The cell was usually round or oval, but occasionally irregular or stellate. The nucleus was generally localized to one pole of the cell and was round or elliptical in shape. Size and location of secretory granules was one of the most useful criteria for identification of gonadotrophs. The granules were round, especially electron opaque and membrane bound . The diameter of one granule type is 150 to 250 nm and that of the other type is 350 to 450 nm. The number of the secretory granules, however, varied widely from one gonadotroph to another, even in the same animal. The Golgi complex occupied much of the cytoplasm in one pole of the cell . A very low, electron-opaque material was observed within Golgi cisternae.

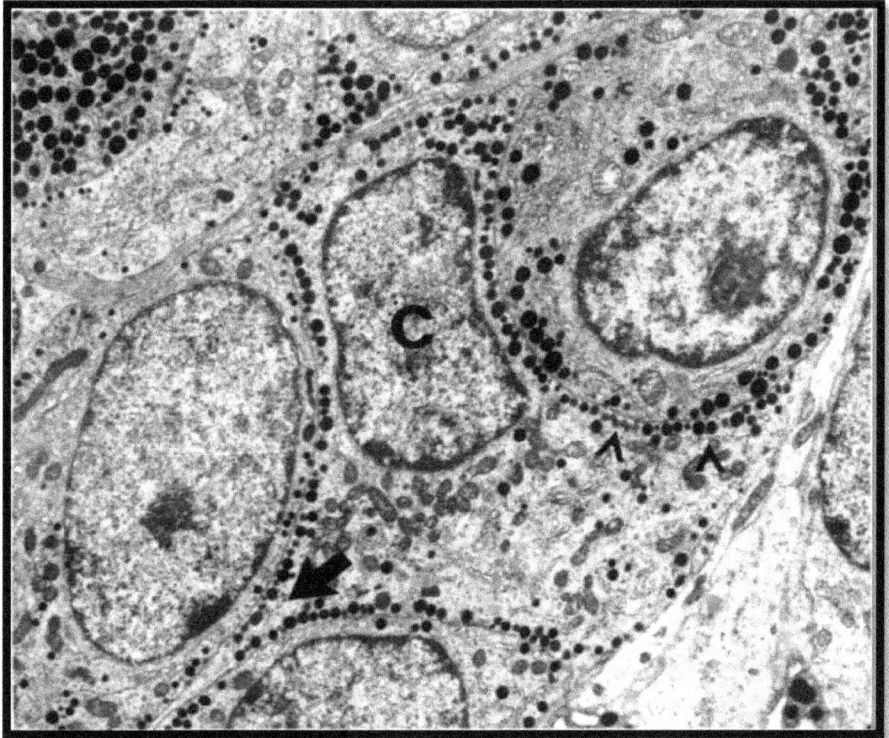

Fig. 84. Normal male rat anterior pituitary (x 6600). Corticotroph (c) showing characteristic stellate shape with processes extending between other cells (~) and peripheral localisation of granules (vv).

Contribution of Scientists

Bernardo Houssay

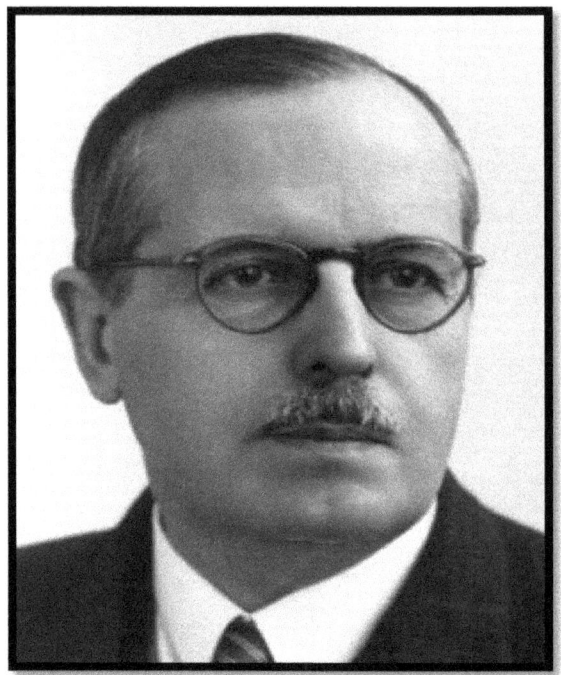

Bernardo Alberto Houssay

The Nobel Prize in Physiology or Medicine 1947
Born: 10 April 1887, Buenos Aires, Argentina
Died: 21 September 1971, Buenos Aires, Argentina
Affiliation at the time of the award:
Instituto de Biologia y Medicina Experimental (Institute for Biology and Experimental Medicine), Buenos Aires, Argentina

Work

For the body to obtain energy, it must be able to convert sugar. The hormone insulin, which is formed in the pancreas, plays an important role in this process. This is also true of the pituitary gland in the brain. In the early 1940s, Bernardo Houssay conducted experiments on dogs and toads to study the pituitary gland's role in this context. After parts of the pituitary were surgically removed from dogs, they became very sensitive to low doses of insulin. This indicated that a hormone is formed in the front portions of the pituitary gland that counteracts and balances the effects of insulin.

CARL FERDINAND CORI

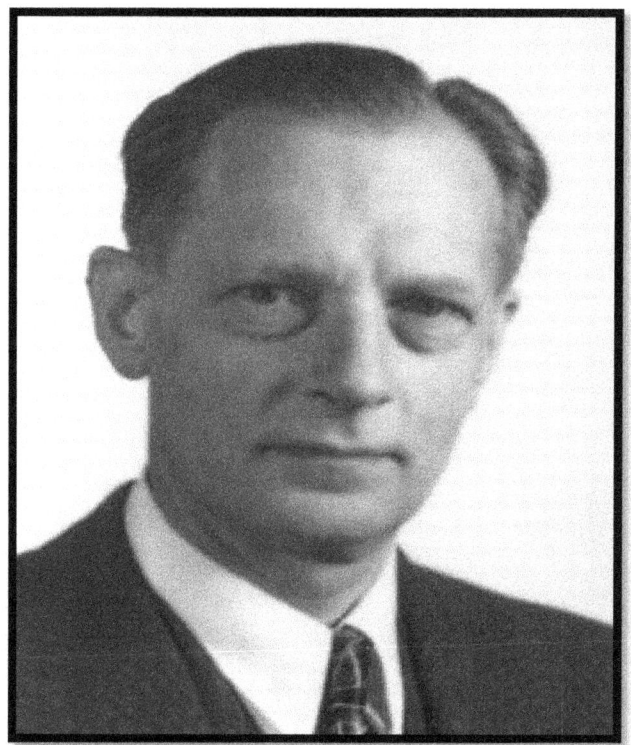

CARL FERDINAND CORI
The Nobel Prize in Physiology or Medicine 1947

Born: 5 December 1896, Prague, Austria-Hungary (now Czech Republic) (now Czechoslovakia)

Died: 20 October 1984, Cambridge, MA, USA

Affiliation at the time of the award : Washington University, St. Louis, MO, USA

Work

Carl and Gerty Cori took an interest in how the body utilizes energy. In 1929, they described what is known as the Cori cycle; an important part of metabolism. Lactic acid forms when we use our muscles, which is then converted into glycogen in the liver. Glycogen, in turn, is converted into glucose, which is absorbed by muscle cells. The pair continued to investigate how glycogen is broken down into glucose and, in 1938-1939, were able to both identify the enzyme that initiates the decomposition and also to use the process to create glycogen in a test tube.

Gerty Theresa Cori, née Radnitz

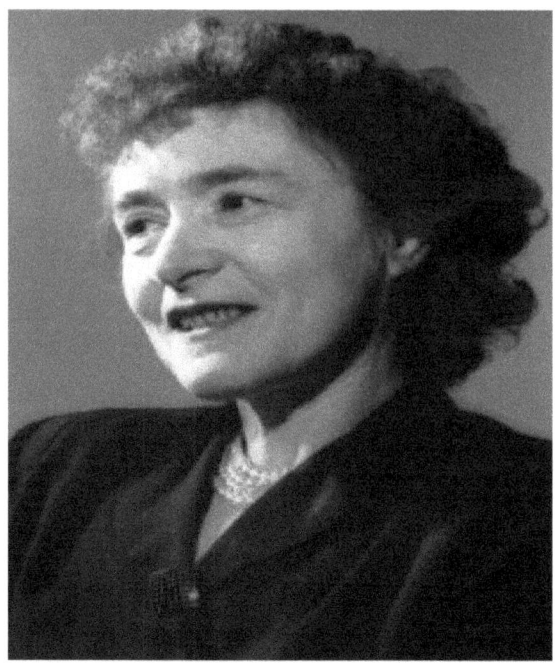

Gerty Theresa Cori, née Radnitz
The Nobel Prize in Physiology or Medicine 1947
Born: 15 August 1896, Prague, Austria-Hungary (now Czech Republic) (now Czechoslovakia)
Died: 26 October 1957, St. Louis, MO, USA
Affiliation at the time of the award: Washington University, St. Louis, MO, USA

Andrew V. Schally

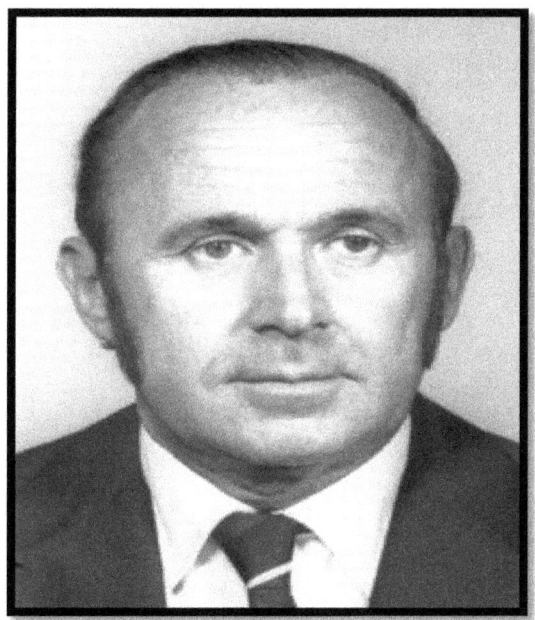

Andrew V. Schally

The Nobel Prize in Physiology or Medicine 1977

Born: 30 November 1926, Wilno (now Vilnius), Poland (now Lithuania)

Affiliation at the time of the award: Veterans Administration Hospital, New Orleans, LA, USA

Work

Hormones are substances that convey signals between different parts of the body and regulate their functions. Around the pituitary in the brain, releasing hormones serve to release other hormones and are formed around the pituitary gland. The releasing hormones occur in very small amounts, from large quantities of pig brains and lamb brains respectively, Andrew Schally and Roger Guillemin separately extracted a sufficient amount of releasing hormone to determine its structure in 1969. They subsequently were able to produce it with chemical methods.

Roger Guillemin

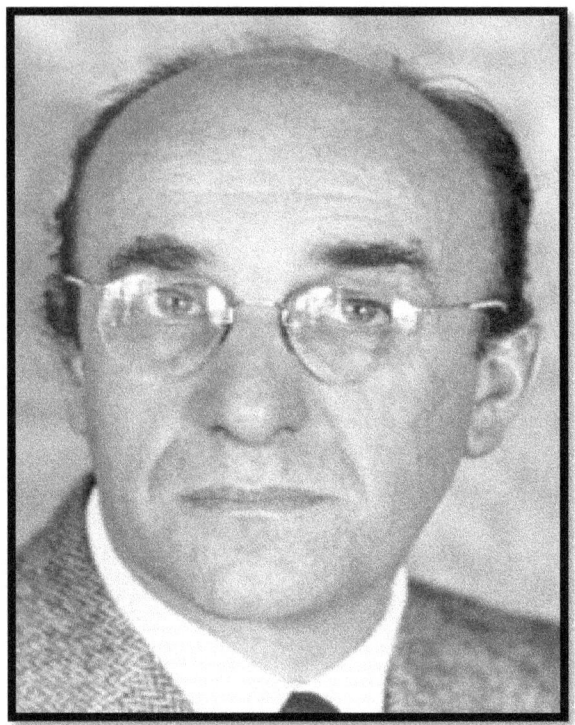

Roger Guillemin

The Nobel Prize in Physiology or Medicine , 1977

Born: 11 January 1924, Dijon, France

Affiliation at the time of the award: The Salk Institute, San Diego, CA, USA

Work

Hormones are substances that convey signals between different parts of the body and regulate their functions. Around the pituitary in the brain, releasing hormones serve to release other hormones and are formed around the pituitary gland. The releasing hormones occur in very small amounts. From large quantities of pig brains and lamb brains respectively, Roger Guillemin and Andrew Schally separately extracted a sufficient amount of releasing hormone to determine its structure in 1969. They subsequently were able to produce it with chemical methods.

Rosalyn Yalow

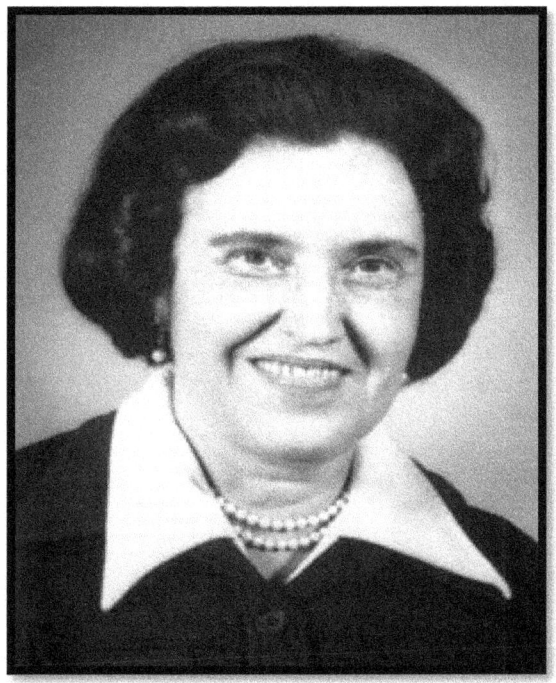

Rosalyn Yalow

The Nobel Prize in Physiology or Medicine 1977

Born: 19 July 1921, New York, NY, USA

Died: 30 May 2011, New York, NY, USA

Affiliation at the time of the award: Veterans Administration Hospital, Bronx, NY, USA

Work

Rosalyn Yalow was a nuclear physicist. She developed radioimmunoassay (RIA) together with Doctor Solomon Berson. RIA is used to measure small concentrations of substances in the body, such as hormones in the blood. Rosalyn Yalow and Solomon Berson tracked insulin by injecting radioactive iodine into patients' blood. Because the method is so precise, they were able to prove that type 2 diabetes is caused by the body's inefficient use of insulin. Previously it was thought that the disease was caused by a lack of insulin.

Solomon Berson

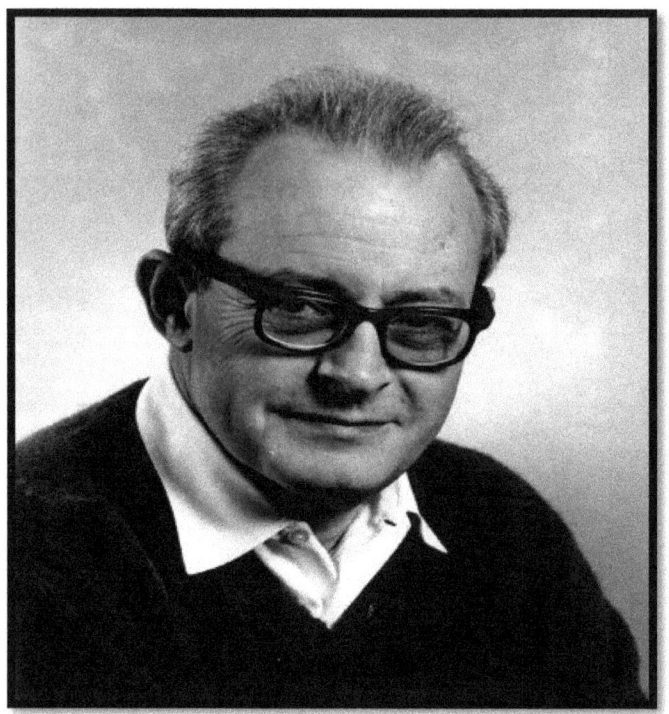

Solomon Berson

Born: April 22, 1918 New York City, New York, U.S.
Died: April 11, 1972 (aged 53) Atlantic City, New Jersey, U.S.
Nationality: American
Occupation: Physician and scientist
Known for: Advances in clinical biochemistry

Scientific career

Berson's scientific work started in 1950, when he became a member of the Radioisotope Service of the hospital, where he teamed with Rosalyn Yalow in what eventually became an historic research partnership. He also set up a thyroid service, where his approach was felt lastingly. Their early laboratory work concerned iodine and human serum albumin metabolism, but later on in the decade they shifted their focus to insulin, a hormone which was difficult to measure in the blood. They developed the radioimmunoassay, which gave very good results, and published their findings in 1960.[They were able to distinguish between two types of diabetes, Type I and Type II, which have significantly different mechanisms.

With the success of the insulin RIA, Berson and Yalow extended their success to other hormones, such as corticotropin, gastrin, parathyroid hormone and growth hormone, making significant discoveries in their physiology along the way.

NEUROHYPOPHYSES

Normal

The posterior pituitary is neural tissue and consists only of the distal axons of the hypothalamic magnocellular neurons that make up the neurohypophysis. The perikarya (cell bodies) of these axons are located in paired paraventricular and supraoptic nuclei of the hypothalamus. During embryogenesis neuroepithelial cells of the lining of the third ventricle mature into magnocellular neurons while migrating laterally to and above the optic chiasm to form the supraoptic nuclei and to the walls of the third ventricle to form the paraventricular nuclei. In the posterior pituitary the axon terminals of the magnocellular neurons contain neurosecretory granules, membrane-bound packets of hormones stored for subsequent release.

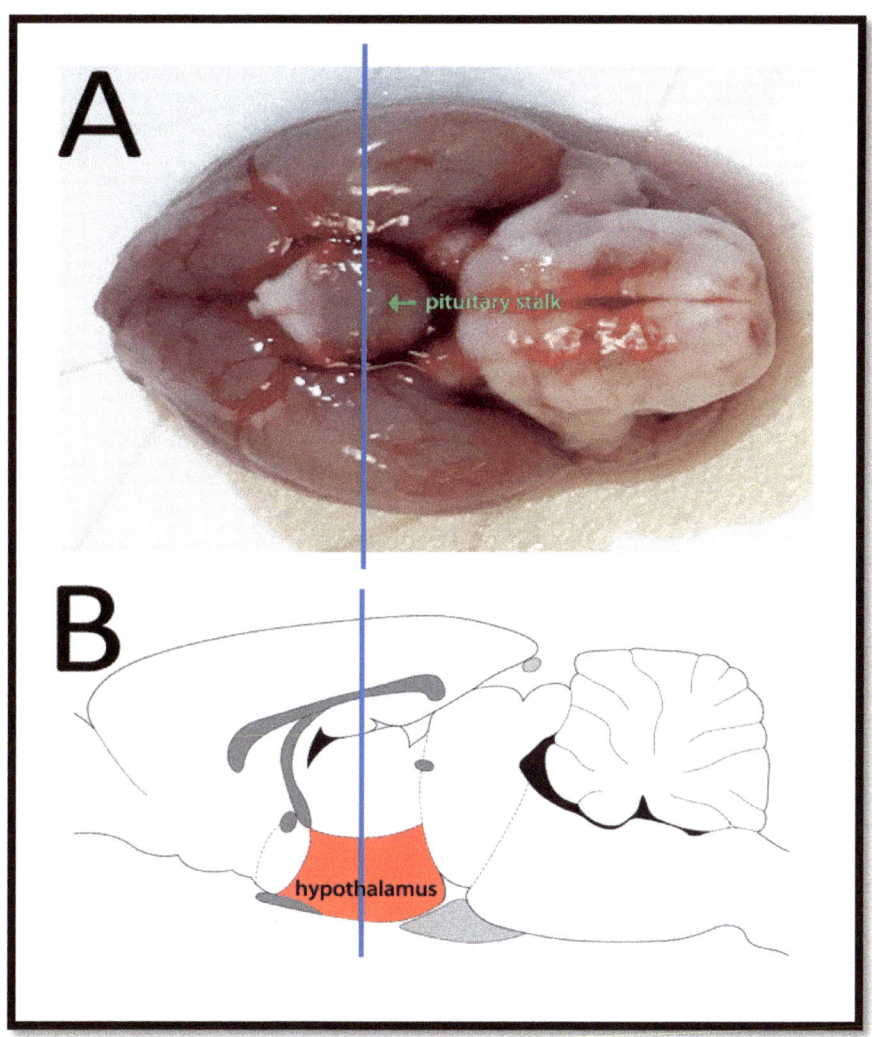

Fig. 85. (A) The inferior view of the rat's brain. (B) the medial view of a saggital section of the rat's brain.

NEUROHYPOPHYSIS (Pars Posterior, Posterior Lobe)

The neurohypophysis does not contain neuroendocrine epithelial cells. Instead, it is composed of the axons arising from groups of hypothalamic neurons, most prominently those originating from magnocellular neurons of the supraoptic and paraventricular nuclei. They form the hypothalamo-hypophyseal tract and their terminals end near the sinusoids of the posterior lobe. The neurosecretory granules mostly contain oxytocin or vasopressin and form axonal beads close to their termini. Whilst it is believed that normal astrocytes may populate (at least partially) the infundibulum, the axon terminals in the neurohypophysis are supported by so-called pituicytes, which are characterised by the expression of the TTF-1 transcription factor (absent in classic GFAP-positive astrocytes). These cells show elongated processes often running in parallel with axons, and demonstrate only patchy GFAP and S100 expression.

Herring bodies or neurosecretory bodies are structures found in the posterior pituitary (neurohypophysis).

They are very large swellings in the axons of the neurosecretory neurons in the posterior pituitary gland and named after Percy Theodore Herring . It represents the terminal end of the axons from the hypothalamus, and hormones such as ADH and Oxytocin are temporarily stored in these locations.

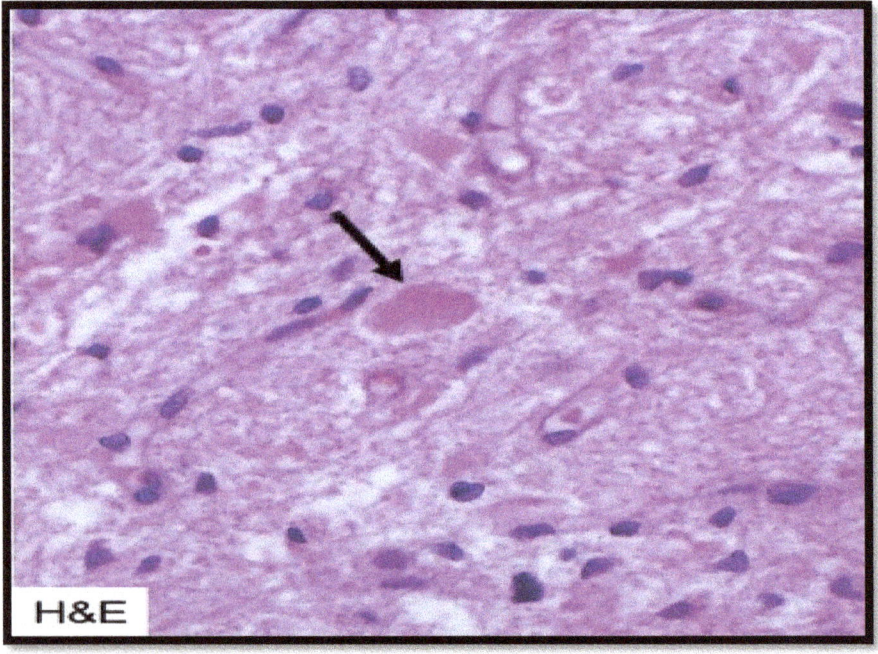

Fig. 86. The cytoarchitecture of the neurophypophysis . The large distended nerve endings can be identified on routine stains as so-called Herring-bodies (arrow), named after Percy Theodore Herring (University of Edinburgh) who described them in 1908 as the 'physiologically active principle' of the posterior gland.

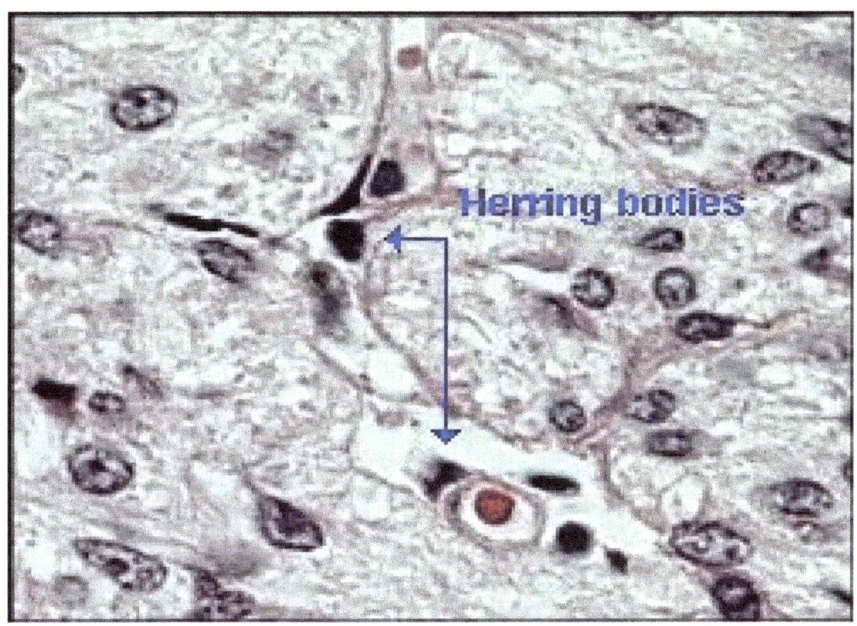

Fig. 87. Histologic feature of the Neurohypophysis

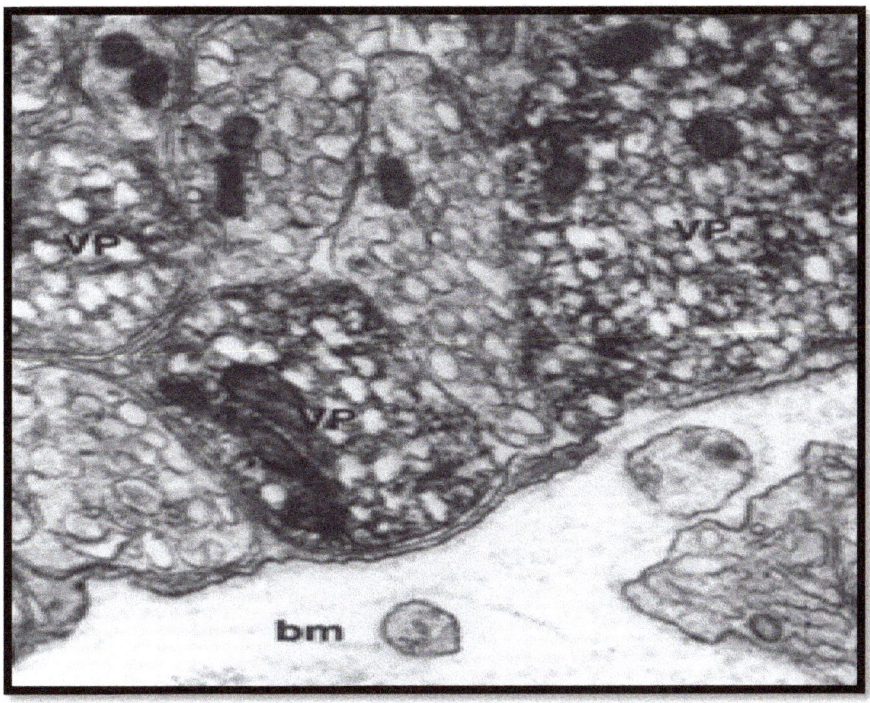

Fig. 88. Control rat. Neurohypophysis. a Mixed VP-labelled (VP) and unlabelled axon profiles filled with NSG. x 21390

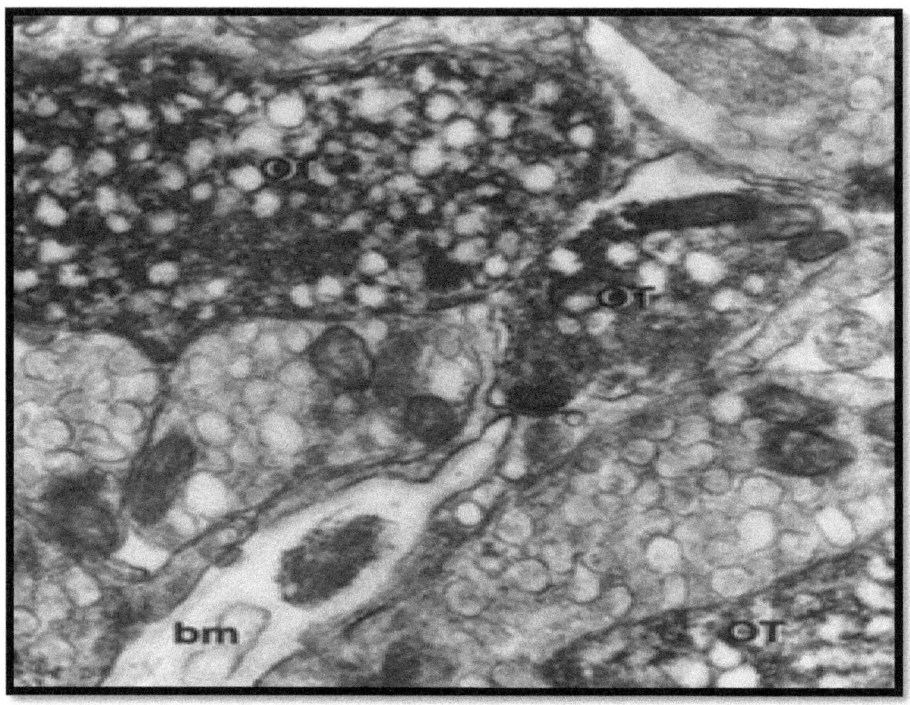

Fig. 89. Mixed OTlabelled (OT) and unlabelled axon profiles filled with NSG. bm: basement membrane, x 25110

Contribution of Scientists

Percy Theodore Herring

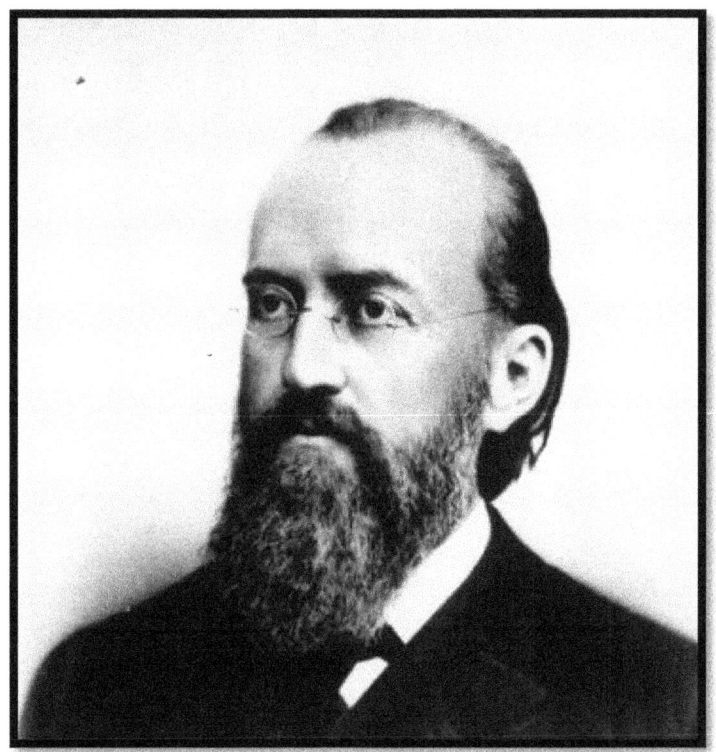

Percy Theodore Herring

Born on November 03, 1872
Died on October 24, 1967.

Percy Theodore Herring was a physician and physiologist notable for first describing Herring bodies in the posterior pituitary gland. He was born in Yorkshire England on 3 November 1872 the son of Edmund Herring and schooled in Christchurch New Zealand. He attended the University of Otago , New Zealand and the University of Edinburgh , Scotland from which he graduated with an MB in 1896.

Awards: Awarded Fellow of the Royal Society of Edinburgh .

CONTRIBUTION

Herring bodies or neurosecretory bodies are structures found in the posterior pituitary. They represent the terminal end of the axons from the hypothalamus, and hormones are temporarily stored in these locations. They are neurosecretory terminals.

Antidiuretic hormone (ADH) and oxytocin are both stored in Herring bodies, but are not stored simultaneously in the same Herring body.

In addition, each Herring body also contains ATP and a type of neurophysin. Neurophysins are binding proteins, of which there are two types: neurophysin I and neurophysin II, which bind to oxytocin and ADH, respectively. Neurophysin and its hormone become a complex considered a single protein and stored in the neurohypophysis. Upon stimulation by the hypothalamus, secretory granules release stored hormones into the bloodstream. Fibers from supraoptic nuclei are concerned with ADH secretion; paraventricular nuclei with oxytocin.

This anatomical structure was first described by Percy Theodore Herring in 1908.

Vincent du Vigneaud

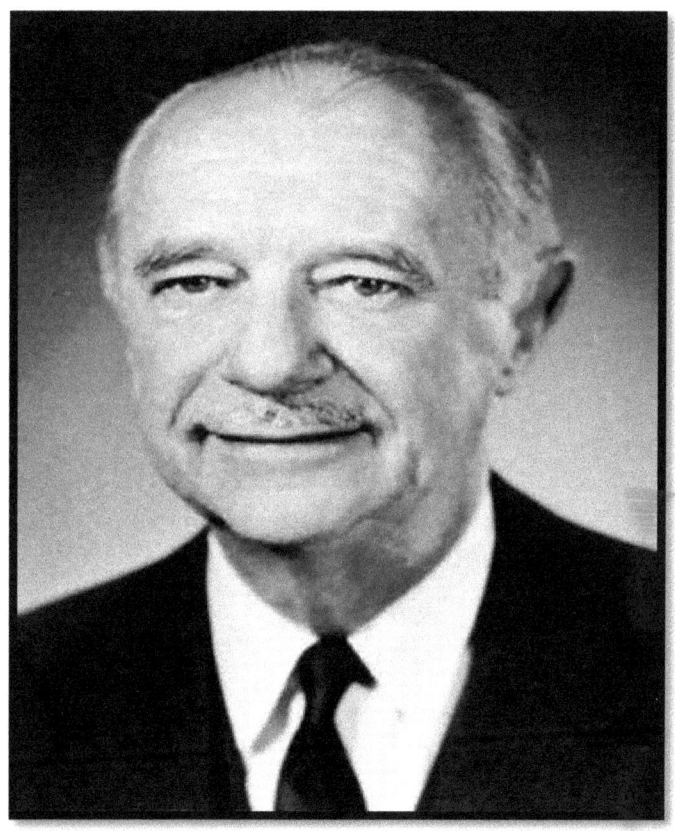

Vincent du Vigneaud
Biochemist
The Nobel Prize in Chemistry 1955
Born: 18 May 1901, Chicago, IL, USA
Died: 11 December 1978, White Plains, NY, USA
Affiliation at the time of the award: Cornell University, Ithaca, NY, USA

CONTRIBUTION

The element sulfur plays an important role in some of the chemical compounds and processes that are the basis of all life. Vincent du Vigneaud studied sulfurous compounds, including oxytocin, a hormone that among other things plays a role in sexual intimacy and reproduction among people and mammals. In 1953 Vincent du Vigneaud succeeded in isolating the substance and determining its chemical composition. It became the first peptide hormone to have its sequence of amino acids determined. He also succeeded in producing oxytocin by artificial means.

Nobel Laureate Dr. Vincent du Vigneaud pioneered research in oxytocin during his long career at Cornell University Medical College (now Weill Cornell Medicine.) Oxytocin, a polypeptide hormone, is responsible for social bonding during sex, childbirth, and breastfeeding. It also produces breast milk and the contractions of the uterus during labor. Dr. du Vigneaud was awarded a Nobel Prize in Chemistry for landmark research in sulfur compounds and the first synthesis of oxytocin in 1955. His work opened new research in the field of protein organic chemistry.

BUFFERS

pH and Buffers Defined

pH is a measure of the concentration of H^+ [H_3O^+] ions in a solution. Only the concentration of H^+ and OH^- molecules determine the pH. When the concentration of H^+ and OH^- ions are equal, the solution is said to be neutral. If there are more H^+ than OH^- molecules the solution is acidic, and if there are more OH^- than H^+ molecules, the solution is basic.

Buffers

To be able to add a strong acid or base to a solution without causing a large change in the pH, we need to create a buffer solution. A buffer solution contains both a weak acid (HA) and its conjugate base (A^-).

Types of buffer solutions:

Acidic buffer

Acid buffer solutions have a pH less than 7. It is generally made from a weak acid and one of its salts (often called conjugate*). Commonly used acidic buffer solutions are a mixture of ethanoic acid and sodium ethanoate in solution, which have a pH of 4.76 when mixed in equal molar concentrations. You can change the pH of the buffer solution by changing the ratio of acid to salt, or by choosing a different acid and one of its salts.

Alkaline buffer

Alkaline buffer solutions have a pH greater than 7 and are made from a weak base and one of its salts. A very commonly used example of an alkaline buffer solution is a mixture of ammonia and ammonium chloride solution. If these were mixed in equal molar proportions, the solution would have a pH of 9.25.

Key Points

- A basic solution will have a pH above 7.0, while an acidic solution will have a pH below 7.0.

- Buffers are solutions that contain a weak acid and its a conjugate base; as such, they can absorb excess H^+ ions or OH^- ions, thereby maintaining an overall steady pH in the solution.
- pH is equal to the negative logarithm of the concentration of H^+ ions in solution: $pH = -\log[H^+]$.

Self-Ionization of Water

Hydrogen ions are spontaneously generated in pure water by the dissociation (ionization) of a small percentage of water molecules into equal numbers of hydrogen **(H^+)** ions and hydroxide (OH^-) ions. The hydroxide ions remain in solution because of their hydrogen bonds with other water molecules; the hydrogen ions, consisting of naked protons, are immediately attracted to un-ionized water molecules and form hydronium ions (H_3O^+). By convention, scientists refer to hydrogen ions and their concentration as if they were free in this state in liquid water.

$$2H_2O \leftrightharpoons H_3O^+ + OH^- - 2H_2O \leftrightharpoons H_3O^+ + OH^-$$

The concentration of hydrogen ions dissociating from pure water is 1×10^{-7} moles H^+ ions per liter of water. The pH is calculated as the negative of the base 10 logarithm of this concentration:

$pH = -\log[H^+]$

The negative log of 1×10^{-7} is equal to 7.0, which is also known as neutral pH. Human cells and blood each maintain near-neutral pH.

pH Scale

The pH of a solution indicates its acidity or basicity (alkalinity). The pH scale is an inverse logarithm that ranges from 0 to 14: anything below 7.0 (ranging from 0.0 to 6.9) is acidic, and anything above 7.0 (from 7.1 to 14.0) is basic (or alkaline). Extremes in pH in either direction from 7.0 are usually considered inhospitable to life. The pH in cells (6.8) and the blood (7.4) are both very close to neutral, whereas the environment in the stomach is highly acidic, with a pH of 1 to 2.

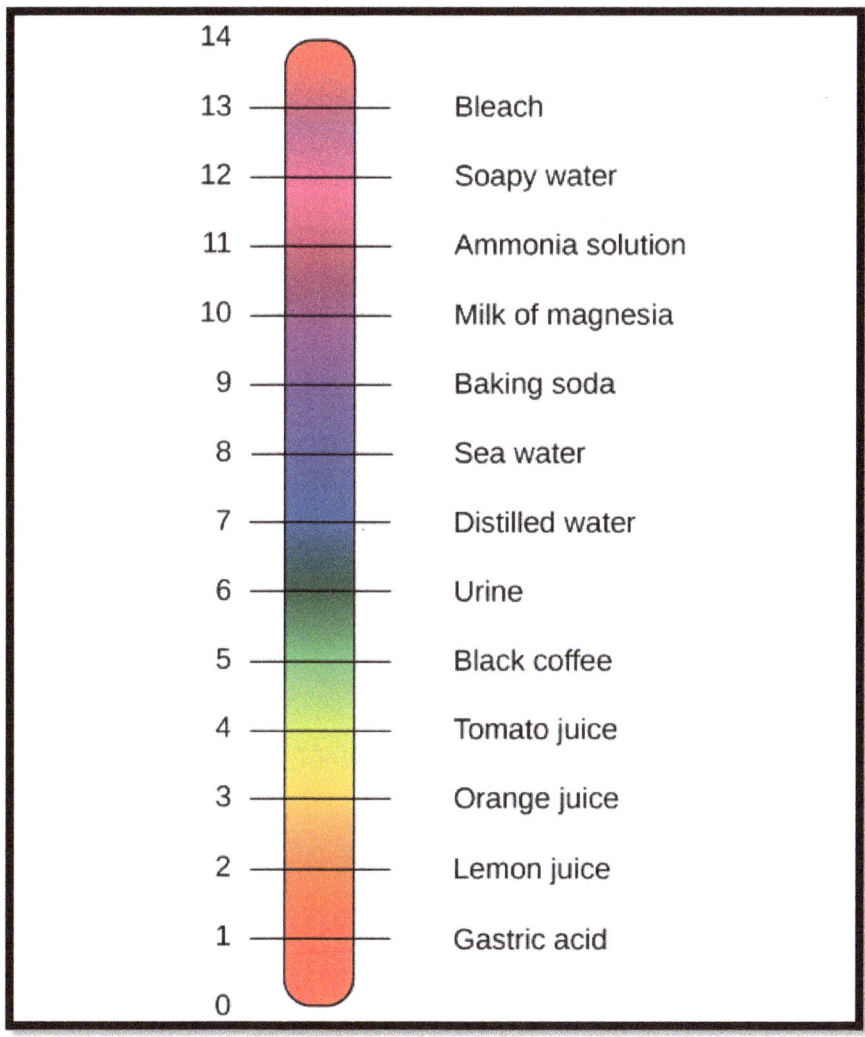

Fig. 90. The pH scale measures the concentration of hydrogen ions (H+) in a solution.

The pH scale : The pH scale measures the concentration of hydrogen ions (H^+) in a solution.

Strong Acids and Strong Bases

The stronger the acid, the more readily it donates H^+. For example, hydrochloric acid (HCl) is highly acidic and completely dissociates into hydrogen and chloride ions, whereas the acids in tomato juice or vinegar do not completely dissociate and are considered weak acids; conversely, strong bases readily donate OH^- and/or react with hydrogen ions. Sodium hydroxide (NaOH) and many household cleaners are highly basic and give up OH^- rapidly when placed in water; the OH^- ions react with H^+ in solution, creating new water molecules and lowering the amount of free H^+ in the system, thereby raising the overall pH. An example of a weak basic solution is seawater, which has a pH near 8.0, close enough to neutral that well-adapted marine organisms thrive in this alkaline environment.

Buffers

How can organisms whose bodies require a near-neutral pH ingest acidic and basic substances (a human drinking orange juice, for example) and survive? Buffers are the key. Buffers usually consist of a weak acid and its conjugate base; this enables them to readily absorb excess H^+ or OH^-, keeping the system's pH within a narrow range.

Maintaining a constant blood pH is critical to a person's well-being. The buffer that maintains the pH of human blood involves carbonic acid (H_2CO_3), bicarbonate ion (HCO_3^-), and carbon dioxide (CO_2). When bicarbonate ions combine with free hydrogen ions and become carbonic acid, hydrogen ions are removed, moderating pH changes. Similarly, excess carbonic acid can be converted into carbon dioxide gas and exhaled through the lungs; this prevents too many free hydrogen ions from building up in the blood and dangerously reducing its pH; likewise, if too much OH^- is introduced into the system, carbonic acid will combine with it to create bicarbonate, lowering the pH. Without this buffer system, the body's pH would fluctuate enough to jeopardize survival.

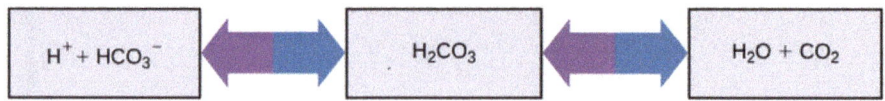

Buffers in the body

This diagram shows the body's buffering of blood pH levels: the blue arrows show the process of raising pH as more CO2 is made; the purple arrows indicate the reverse process, lowering pH as more bicarbonate is created.

Antacids, which combat excess stomach acid, are another example of buffers. Many over-the-counter medications work similarly to blood buffers, often with at least one ion (usually carbonate) capable of absorbing hydrogen and moderating pH, bringing relief to those that suffer "heartburn" from stomach acid after eating.

Choice of Buffers during fixation

The quality of fixation is influenced by pH and the type of ions present.

The choice of buffer is based on:
1. the buffering capacity in the desired pH range with the ability to maintain constant pH during fixation.
2. the side effects which vary with the tissue type:
    a) suitable osmolarity so that cells and organelles neither swell nor shrink during fixation.
    b) suitable ionic concentration so that materials are neither extracted nor precipitated during fixation.
    c) the toxicity of the buffer.

Criteria of a good buffer:

1. **pKa** : usually between 6 and 8 desired for biological specimens.
2. Maximum solubility in water and minimum solubility in all other solvents.
3. Reduced ion effects.
4. Dissociation of buffer least influenced by buffer concentration, temperature and ionic composition.
5. Resistance to oxidation (stable).
6. Inexpensive and easy to prepare.
7. No reaction with fixation.

Common Buffers

Phosphate Buffer (Sorenson's buffer) pH 5.8-8

Advantages:
1. Most physiological of common buffers. Mimics certain components of extracellular fluids.
2. Non-toxic to cells.
3. pH changes little with temperature.
4. Stable for several weeks at 4 C.

Disadvantages:
1. Precipitates more likely to occur during fixation. Tends to form precipitates in presence of calcium ions. Precipitates uranyl acetate and tends to react with lead salts.
2. Becomes slowly contaminated with micro-organisms

Preparation of Buffer

Stock solutions:

0.2M dibasic sodium phosphate 1 liter

$Na_2HPO_4 * 2H_2O$	(MW = 178.05)	35.61 gm
or		
$Na_2HPO_4 * 7H_2O$	(MW = 268.07)	53.65 gm
or		
$Na_2HPO_4 * 12H_2O$	(MW = 358.14)	71.64 gm
+ ddH$_2$0 to make		1 liter

0.2M monobasic sodium phosphate 1 litter

$NaH_2PO_4 * H_2O$	(MW = 138.01)	27.6 gm
or		
$NaH_2PO_4 * 2H_2O$	(MW = 156.03)	31.21 gm
+ ddH$_2$0 to make		1 liter

Working buffer: 0.1M 100 ml

Mix X ml of **0.2M dibasic sodium phosphate** with Y ml **monobasic sodium phosphate.** Dilute to 100 ml with ddH$_2$0 or dilute 1:1 with fixative.

pH(25C)	Xml	Yml
5.8	4.0	46.0
6.0	6.15	43.75
6.2	9.25	40.75
6.4	13.25	36.75
6.6	18.75	31.25
6.8	24.5	25.5
7.0	30.5	19.5
7.2	36.0	14.0
7.4	40.5	9.5
7.6	43.5	6.5
7.8	45.75	4.25
8.0	47.35	2.65

Osmolarity is adjusted by varying the molarity of phosphates or by the addition of sucrose, glucose or sodium chloride.

At pH 7.2 :

0.10M = 226 mOs (milliosmoles)
0.05M = 118 mOs
0.075 = 180 mOs
0.15M = 350 mOs

II. Cacodylate Buffer (arsenate buffer) pH 5 - 7.4

Advantages:
1. Easy to prepare.
2. Stable during storage for long periods of time.
3. Does not support growth of microorganisms.

5. Precipitates usually do not occur. Precipitates do not occur at low concentrations of calcium.

Disadvantages:
1. Toxic. Contains arsenic.
2. Unpleasant smell.

Preparation of Buffer:
Stock solutions:
    0.2M sodium cacodylate 1 liter

$Na(CH_3)_2AsO_2 * 3H_2O$	(MW = 195.92)	42.8 gm
+ ddH_2O to make	1 liter	

0.2M HCl
Conc. HCl (36-38%)	10 ml
ddH_2O	603 ml

Working buffer: 0.1M   100 ml

Adjust 50 ml of 0.2M sodium cacodylate to desired pH with 0.2M HCl. Dilute to 100 ml with ddH_2O or dilute 1:1 with fixative.

pH	0.2M HCl (ml)
6.4	18.3
6.6	13.3
6.8	9.3
7.0	6.3
7.2	4.2
7.4	2.7

Buffer may also be made with cacodylic acid.

Stock solutions:
    0.2M cacodylic acid 1 liter

$(CH_3)_2AsO_2H$	(MW = 138.0)	27.6 gm
+ ddH$_2$0 to make		1 liter

0.2M NaOH   100 ml

NaOH	(MW = 40)	0.8 gm
+ ddH$_2$0 to make		100 ml

Working buffer: 0.1M
Adjust 50 ml of 0.2M cacodylic acid to desired pH with 0.2M NaOH. Dilute to 100 ml with ddH$_2$ or dilute 1:1 with fixative.

III. Veronal-acetate Buffer (Michaelis buffer)

Advantages:
Useful for block staining with uranyl acetate since precipitates do not form.

Disadvantages:
1. Reacts with aldehydes.
2. Poor buffer at physiological pH.
3. Supports growth of micro-organisms.
4. Contains barbiturate.

Preparation of Buffer:
Stock solution: 0.28M   100 ml
   Sodium veronal (barbitone sodium)

$C_8H_{11}0_3N_2Na$	(MW = 206.18)	2.89 gm

   Sodium acetate (anhydrous)

CH_3C00Na	(MW = 82.03)	1.15 gm

or
   Sodium acetate (hydrated)

$CH_3C00Na*3H_20$	(MW = 136.09)	1.90 gm
+ ddH$_2$H$_2$0 to make		100 ml

   Solution is stable and may be stored for some months at 4 C.

Working buffer:
Veronal acetate stock solution	5 ml

ddH$_2$0   15 ml

Add 0.1 HCl gradually to desired pH.

Solution cannot be stored.

> Supports growth of bacteria and molds even at 4 C.
> Crystallizes in absence of osmium tetroxide.

IV. Collidine Buffer   pH 7.25-7.74

Advantages:
1. Maximum buffering capacity about 7.4.
2. Stable indefinitely at room temperature.
3. Useful for fixation of large tissue blocks. Aids penetration of fixative due to extractive effects (see disadvantage 1).

Disadvantages:
4. Not suitable as buffer during primary fixation with osmium tetroxide due to considerable extraction of tissue components.
5. Use leads to lysis of cytoplasmic matrix and extensive membrane destruction when used with paraformaldehyde fixatives.
6. Use gives poorer results with glutaraldehyde than those obtained with phosphate or cacodylate buffer.

Preparation of Buffer:

Stock solution: 0.4M   100 ml
    Pure s-collidine   5.34 gm
    2,4,6(CH$_3$)$_3$(C$_2$H$_5$N)   (MW = 121.18)
    + ddH$_2$0 to make   100 ml

Working buffer: 0.2M   100 ml

Adjust 50 ml of s-collidine stock solution to desired pH with 1N HCl. Dilute to 100 ml with ddH$_2$0.

pH	1N HCl (ml)
7.25	22
7.33	20
7.41	18

7.5	16
7.59	14
7.67	12
7.74	10

V. Tris buffer

Advantages:
1. Good buffering capacity at higher pH required for some tissues and some cytochemical procedures.
2. "More or less" physiologically inert.

Disadvantages:
1. pH changes with temperature. Must be measured at desired temperature.
2. pH must be measured with certain type of electrode.

Preparation of Buffer:
   A. Tris Buffer   pH 7.1-8.9
   Stock solution   0.2M   1 liter
      Tris(hydroxymethyl)aminomethane   24.2 gm
        $H_2NC(CH_2OH)_3$ (MW = 121.13)
      + ddH_2O to make   1 liter

Working buffer: 0.1M   100 ml
Adjust pH of 50 ml of stock solution with 0.1M NaOH. Dilute to 100 ml with ddH_2O.

   B. Tris-maleate Buffer   pH 5.8-8.2
   Stock solution: 0.2M   liter
      Tris(hydroxymethyl)aminomethane   24.2 gm
      Maleic acid   23.2 gm
        $HO_2CCH{:}CHCO_2H$ (MW = 116.07)
      + ddH_2O to make   1 liter
  or
      Trizima-maleate   (MW = 237.2)   47.4 gm

+ ddH₂0 to make   1 liter

Working buffer: 0.2M   100 ml
Adjust 50 ml of stock solution to desired pH with 0.1M NaOH. Dilute to 100 ml with ddH₂0.

VI. Special Buffers Used for Cytochemical Reactions.

A. **Acetate Buffer**   (sodium acetate-acetic acid buffer) pH 4-5.6
Sodium acetate   0.2M = 27.2 gm/l
$CH_3CO_2Na*3H_2O$ (MW - 136.09)
Acetic acid   0.2M
CH_3COOH (MW = 60)
Add sodium acetate to acetic acid to give desired pH. Dilute with ddH₂0 to desired molarity.

B. **Borate Buffer**   pH 7.4-9.2
Borax (sodium tetraborate)   0.2M = 76.2 gm/ml
$Na_2B_4O_7*120H_2O$ (MW = 381.37)
Boric acid   0.2M = 12.37 gm/l
H_3BO_3 (MW = 61.83)
Add boric acid to borax solution until desired pH is reached. Dilute to desired molarity with ddH₂0.

C. **Citrate Buffer** (sodium citrate-citric acid buffer) pH 3-6.2
Sodium citrate   0.2M = 58.8 gm/l
$Na_3C_6H_5O_7*H_2O$ (MW = 294.12)
Citric acid   0.2M = 42.02 gm/l
$C_6H_8O_7*H_2O$ (MW = 210.14)
Mix citric acid and sodium citrate to give desired pH. Dilute with ddH₂0 to desired molarity.

D. **Dimethylglutarate Buffer**   pH 3.2-7.6
Dimethylglutaric acid   0.1M = 16.02 gm/l
$C_7H_{12}O_4$ (MW = 160.2)

Add 0.2N NaOH to give desired pH. Dilute with ddH$_2$O to desired molarity.

E. **Succinate Buffer**   pH 3.8-6
Succinic acid   0.2M = 23/62 g/l
C$_4$H$_6$O$_2$ (MW = 118.09)
Add 0.2M NaOH to desired pH. Dilute with ddH$_2$O to desired molarity.

F. **Maleate Buffer** (sodium hydrogen maleate buffer) pH 5.2-6.8
Stock solution: 0.2M 1 liter
Maleic acid (MW = 121.14)   23.2 gm
+ ddH$_2$O to make   1 liter
Adjust pH with 0.1M NaOH. Dilute with ddH$_2$O to desired molarity.

G. **Imidazole Buffer** pH 6.2-7.8
Imidazole   0.2M = 13.62/1
C$_3$H$_4$N$_2$ (MW = 68.08)
Adjust 0.2N HCl to imidazole solution until desired pH is reached. Dilute to desired molarity with ddH$_2$O.

H. **AMPd Buffer**   pH 7.8-9.7
2-amino-methyl-1,3-propanediol   0.2M = 21.03 gm/l
C$_4$H$_{11}$NO$_2$ (MW = 105.14)
Add 0.2M HCl until desired pH is reached. Dilute with ddH$_2$O to desired molarity.

Common Biological Buffers

The following are recipes for a number of common biological buffers taken from *Ruzin, 1999 Plant Microtechnique and Microscopy*. When choosing one for a particular application select a buffer based on its pH optimum and biological properties rather than its historical use. Many buffer species have an impact on biological systems, enzyme activities, substrates, or cofactors (Perrin and Dempsey, 1974). For example, phosphate buffers inhibit the activity of several metabolic enzymes including carboxylase, fumarase, and phosphoglucomutase. Barbiturate uncouples oxidative phosphorylation. Tris buffer reacts with primary amines and modifies electron transport and phosphorylation in chloroplasts. Tris also inhibits respiratory enzymes in mitochondria. HEPES does not have these negative effects yet buffers at a similar pH range. MOPS and MES decompose when autoclaved in the presence of glucose. Keep buffer concentration as low as possible yet enough to maintain pH.

GLYCINE–HCL; PH 2.2–3.6, $PK_A = 2.35$

Combine 25 ml 0.2 M glycine and x ml HCl and dilute to 100 ml with DI (Dawson, *et al.*, 1969).

x (ml)	pH
22.0	2.2
16.2	2.4
12.1	2.6
8.4	2.8
5.7	3.0
4.1	3.2
3.2	3.4
2.5	3.6

SODIUM ACETATE; PH 3.6–5.6, $PK_A = 4.76$

Combine the following proportions of $0.1N$ acetic acid and $0.1N$ sodium acetate (Pearse, 1980).

acetic acid	sodium acetate	pH
185	15	3.6
176	24	3.8
164	36	4.0
147	53	4.2
126	74	4.4
102	98	4.6
80	120	4.8
59	141	5.0
42	158	5.2
29	171	5.4
19	181	5.6

BUFFERED SALINE (PBS, TBS, TNT, PBT)

Buffered saline solutions are used frequently when performing immunolocalization experiments. There are many variations. Presented here are three common formulations (Mishkind, *et al.*, 1987).

PBS 20x stock			TBS
Potassium chloride	4 g	53.6 mM	Potassium chloride 4 g
NaCl	160 g	274 mM	NaCl 160 g
Potassium phosphate monobasic	4 g	29.4 mM	Tris buffer (10 mM, pH 7.5) to 1 liter
Sodium phosphate dibasic (7•H2O) DI	43.2 g	17.5 mM to 1 liter	Use TBS when performing immunocytochemical experiments on phosphate-sensitive tissues (photosynthetic tissues typically)
TNT			PBT

NaCl	150 mM	PBS to vol
Tris buffer (100 mM, to pH 7.5)	1 liter	Tween 20 1% (v/v)

CACODYLATE BUFFER; PH 5.0–7.4, PK$_A$ = 6.27

Sodium cacodylate buffer [Na(CH3)2 AsO2 • 3H2O] is a alternative to Sørensen's phosphate buffer. It has good pH buffering capacity within the range of pH 5.0–7.4. Cacodylate was introduced for electron microscopy applications by Sabatini *et al.* (1962) as a method of avoiding adding additional phosphates to sample preparations. Mitochondria and other organelles can be damaged when exposed to the high concentrations of phosphates present in Sørensen's buffers. Also, cacodylate will not react with aldehyde fixatives as will amine-containing buffers (*e.g.,* Tris). Its efficacy in fixation solutions may be a result of the metabolism-inhibiting effect of the arsenate rather than any special buffering capacity.

Prepare a 0.2 M stock solution of sodium cacodylate in water (4.28 g/100 ml). Add the following amounts of 0.2 M HCl per 100 ml cacodylate stock solution, followed by the addition of DI to a final volume of 400 ml, to obtain 0.05 M cacodylate buffer at the desired pH (Dawes, 1971).

0.2 M HCl	pH
94.0	5.0
90.0	5.2
86.0	5.4
78.4	5.6
69.6	5.8
59.2	6.0
47.6	6.2
36.6	6.4
26.6	6.6
18.6	6.8
12.6	7.0
8.4	7.2
5.4	7.4

"GOOD" BUFFERS; PK_A = 6.15–8.06

Tris–HCl (pKa = 8.06) and maleate (pKa = 6.26) have a working range of pH 5.0–8.6 and may be used successfully to buffer staining solutions (*e.g.,* Toluidine Blue O). Avoid Tris with aldehyde fixatives or osmium tetroxide, however, as the aldehydes reacts with the amino group of Tris, resulting in the loss of buffering capacity. PIPES (pKa = 6.80) is commonly used as a buffer for retention of actin filaments during fixation. Other useful biological buffers include HEPES (pKa = 7.55), MES (pKa = 6.15), and MOPS (pKa = 7.20) (Good, *et al.*, 1966; Perrin and Dempsey, 1974).

CITRATE BUFFER; PH 3.0–6.2, PK_A = 6.40 Citrate buffer (Gomori, 1955) stock solutions: **A**: 0.1 M citric acid; **B**: 0.1 M sodium citrate. Use x ml A + y ml B and dilute to 100 ml with 50 ml DI.

0.1 M citric acid	0.1 M sodium citrate	pH
46.5	3.5	3.0
43.7	6.3	3.2
40.0	10.0	3.4
37.0	13.0	3.6
35.0	15.0	3.8
33.0	17.0	4.0
31.5	18.5	4.2
28.0	22.0	4.4
25.5	24.5	4.6
23.0	27.0	4.8
20.5	29.5	5.0
18.0	32.0	5.2
16.0	34.0	5.4
13.7	36.3	5.6
11.8	38.2	5.8
9.5	41.5	6.0
7.2	42.8	6.2

SØRENSEN'S PHOSPHATE BUFFER; PH 5.8–8.0, $PK_A = 7.20$

Mix appropriate volumes of stock and add an equal volume of distilled water to make a final 0.1 M Sørensen's phosphate buffer solution (Sørensen, 1909; Gomori, 1955). Keep in mind that high levels of phosphate may be somewhat toxic to plant cells (Sabatini, *et al.*, 1962) and thus Sørensen's buffer may not be appropriate for some experiments.

Stock solutions: **A** 0.2 M NaH_2PO_4 **B** 0.2 M Na_2HPO_4

A (ml)	B (ml)	pH
92.0	8.0	5.8
87.7	12.3	6.0
81.5	18.5	6.2
68.5	31.5	6.5
62.5	37.5	6.6
56.5	43.5	6.7
51.0	49.0	6.8
45.0	55.0	6.9
39.0	61.0	7.0
33.0	67.0	7.1
28.0	72.0	7.2
23.0	77.0	7.3
19.0	81.0	7.4
16.0	84.0	7.5
8.5	91.5	7.8
5.3	94.7	8.0

PHOSPHATE–CITRATE BUFFER; PH 2.2–8.0, PK_A = 7.20/6.40

Add the following to create 100 ml of phosphate/citrate buffer solution. Stock solutions are

0.2 M dibasic sodium phosphate; 0.1 M citric acid (Pearse, 1980).

0.2 M Na_2HPO_4 (ml)	0.1 M citrate (ml)	pH

5.4	44.6	2.6
7.8	42.2	2.8
10.2	39.8	3.0
12.3	37.7	3.2
14.1	35.9	3.4
16.1	33.9	3.6
17.7	32.3	3.8
19.3	30.7	4.0
20.6	29.4	4.2
22.2	27.8	4.4
23.3	26.7	4.6
24.8	25.2	4.8
25.7	24.3	5.0
26.7	23.3	5.2
27.8	22.2	5.4
29.0	21.0	5.6
30.3	19.7	5.8
32.1	17.9	6.0
33.1	16.9	6.2
34.6	15.4	6.4
36.4	13.6	6.6
40.9	9.1	6.8
43.6	6.5	7.0

BARBITAL BUFFER; PH 6.8–9.2, PK$_A$ = 7.98

Add the following to create 200 ml of buffered solution. To 50 ml of 0.2 M sodium barbital (Veronal, 41.2 g in 1000 ml) add x ml 0.2 M HCl to create the buffered solution and dilute to 200 ml with DI (Gomori, 1955).

0.2 M HCl (ml)	pH

1.5	9.2
2.5	9.0
4.0	8.8
6.0	8.6
9.0	8.4
12.7	8.2
17.5	8.0
22.5	7.8
27.5	7.6
32.5	7.4
39.0	7.2
43.0	7.0
45.0	6.8

TRIS BUFFERS

Tris buffers are used commonly in microtechnique applications involving molecular biological procedures. Listed here are a number of common Tris formulations (Maniatis, *et al.*, 1982).

Solution	Preparation
Tris, 1 M stock	Tris base DI Dissolve and adjust pH with the following approximate amount of HCl: pH 7.4 pH 7.6 pH 8.0 121.1 g 800 ml 70 ml 60 ml 42 ml
EDTA, 0.5 M	Disodium ethylene diamine tetraacetate 186.1 g Adjust pH to approx. 8.0 and stir until dissolved
SSC, 20x	NaCl NaCitrate DI Adjust pH to 7.0 with NaOH then add DI to 1 liter 175.3 g 88.2 g 800 ml

SSPE, 20x	NaCl NaH2PO4 • H2O EDTA DI Adjust pH to 7.4 with NaOH then add DI to 1 liter	174 g 27.6 g 7.4 g 800 ml
TE	Tris EDTA Adjust pH using Tris stock solution	10 mM 1 mM
STE (TNE)	Tris NaCl EDTA Adjust pH to 8.0 using Tris stock solution	10 mM 100 mM 1 mM

GLYCINE– NAOH BUFFER; PH 8.6–10.6, PK$_A$ = 9.78

Stock solutions:

0.2 M glycine
0.2 NaOH

Combine 25 ml glycine stock solution with x ml 0.2 M NaOH and dilute with DI to make a 100 ml solution (Pearse, 1980).

0.2 M NaOH	pH
2.0	8.6
3.0	8.8
4.4	9.0
6.0	9.2
8.4	9.4
11.2	9.6
13.6	9.8
19.3	10.4
22.75	10.6

Preparation of McIlvaine buffer requires disodium phosphate and citric acid. One liter of 0.2M stock solution of disodium phosphate can be prepared by dissolving 28.38g of disodium phosphate in water, and adding a quantity of water sufficient to make one liter. One liter of 0.1M stock solution of citric acid can be prepared by dissolving 19.21g of citric acid in water, and adding a quantity of water sufficient to make one liter. From these stock solutions, McIlvaine buffer can be prepared in accordance with the following table:

Mixing table for obtaining 20 mL of McIlvaine buffer

pH	0.2 M Na_2HPO_4 (mL)	0.1 M citric acid (mL)
2.2	00.40	19.60
2.4	01.24	18.76
2.6	02.18	17.82
2.8	03.17	16.83
3.0	04.11	15.89
3.2	04.94	15.06
3.4	05.70	14.30
3.6	06.44	13.56
3.8	07.10	12.90
4.0	07.71	12.29
4.2	08.28	11.72
4.4	08.82	11.18
4.6	09.35	10.65
4.8	09.86	10.14
5.0	10.30	09.70
5.2	10.72	09.28
5.4	11.15	08.85
5.6	11.60	08.40
5.8	12.09	07.91
6.0	12.63	07.37

Mixing table for obtaining 20 mL of McIlvaine buffer

pH	0.2 M Na_2HPO_4 (mL)	0.1 M citric acid (mL)
6.2	13.22	06.78
6.4	13.85	06.15
6.6	14.55	05.45
6.8	15.45	04.55
7.0	16.47	03.53
7.2	17.39	02.61
7.4	18.17	01.83
7.6	18.73	01.27
7.8	19.15	00.85
8.0	19.45	00.55

Relation between molarity and molality

The composition of a solution is described by the term 'Concentration'. Now, it depends on us whether we define it quantitatively or qualitatively. Like if we define it qualitatively, we would say that the solution is either dilute (less quantity of solute is present) or concentrated (more quantity of solute is present).

But there's a problem in defining the concentration of a solution qualitatively, like what should be the minimum amount of solute for the solution to be called the concentrated or maximum amount of solute present in the solution for it to be called dilute.

So, in order to solve this problem, we have to define concentration quantitatively. For example, molarity and molality are two concentration terms.

MOLARITY – It is defined as the number of moles of solute per litre of the solution.

$$Molarity = \frac{\text{number of moles of the solute}}{\text{volume of the solution(in litres)}}$$

MOLALITY – It is defined as the number of moles of solute per kilogram of the solvent.

$$Molality = \frac{\text{number of moles of solute}}{\text{mass of the solvent(in kg)}}$$

Relation between molarity and molality

We know that $molarity(C) = \frac{\text{number of moles of the solute}}{\text{volume of the solution(in litres)}} = \frac{a}{V}$ ----(1)

a = number of moles of solute
V = volume of solution in a litre

$$molality(m) = \frac{\text{number of moles of solute}}{\text{mass of the solvent(in kg)}} = \frac{a}{W1}$$

m = molality
a = number of moles of solute
W_1 = mass of solvent
Therefore, a = m(W_1) -----(2)

Putting (2) in (1), we get

$$C = \frac{m W_1}{V} \quad ----(3)$$

W_1 = (mass of solution) – (mass of solute)
$$\Rightarrow W_1 = d \times V - a \times \frac{M}{1000} \quad ----(4)$$

Where M = molar mass of solute
d = density of the solution

Putting (4) in (3), we get

$$C = \frac{m}{V d \times V - a \times \frac{M}{1000}}$$

$$m = \frac{C \times V d \times V - a \times M}{1000}$$

$$m = \frac{C \times V V d - a \times M 1000}{V}$$

Now putting $a/V = C$ in the above equation
$$m = \frac{C \times 1}{d - C \times \frac{M}{1000}}$$

$$m = \frac{1000 C}{1000 d - C \times M}$$

Where C = molarity
d = density of solution
M = molar mass of solute

Some questions on molarity and molality

Q1) Why molality is preferred over molarity?
Molality is defined as the number of moles of solutes that are present in 1kg solvent. We know that mass is independent of temperature. Therefore, if there is any change in temperature, then molality remains the same. This is why molality has a preference over molarity.

Q2) What are the S.I. units of molarity and molality?
Molarity is the number of moles of solute per litre of solution. Therefore, its S.I. unit is **mol/lt**. Whereas molality is the number of moles of solute per kg of solvent, therefore, S.I. unit of molality is **mol/kg**.

Q3) Which has more concentration: 1M or 1m?

1M means 1 molar solution, which contains 1 mole of solute in a 1-litre solution and that 1-litre solution consists of both solute and solvent. On the other hand, 1m means 1 molal solution, which contains 1 mole of solute in 1 kg of solvent, which is around 1-litre solvent. Now, we can clearly see that 1m solution contains more quantity of solvent as compared to 1M solution, and both has 1-mole solute. Therefore, 1M has more concentration as compared to 1m.

Q4) How molarity is dependent on temperature?

We know that molarity is the number of moles of solute per litre of solution, and when we increase the temperature, we also have an increase in volume. Therefore, the molarity decreases, and this way, molarity is dependent on temperature.

Q5) Which of the following depends on pressure: molality or molarity?

Molality depends only on the mass of the solvent, but molarity is dependent on the volume of solution, and volume can be changed through a change in pressure and temperature. Also, therefore unlike molality, molarity is dependent on pressure.

Q6) If we are working with a range of temperatures, then which is more preferable: molality or molarity?

We know that molality does not change with a change in temperature. Therefore, molality will be more convenient to use when working with a range of temperatures.

Q7) Which is the S.I. unit of mole fraction?

This is unitless because it is the ratio of moles to moles which too are individually unitless.

Q8) What is normality?

Normality is also a way that is used to calculate the concentration of a solution. It is equal to the gm equivalent weight of solute per litre of the solution. Its S.I. unit is eq/lt. 'N' stands for normality.

Q9) What do you mean by 1 to 3 dilution?

1:3 dilution means that you have 1 unit volume of solute and 3 unit volume of solvent, and when both are combined, then a solution of 4 unit volume is produced.

Q10) What is meant by 2% w/w and 5% w/v solution?

2% w/w - It means that in 100 grams solution, 2 grams of solute is present.

5% w/v – It means that in 100 ml of solution, there is 5 grams of solute.

Molarity of Concentrated Acids & Bases

【Quick reference chart of common acid and base concentrations】

Compound	Molecular formula	Molecular weight	Purity (w/w%)	Specific gravity (20°C)	Concentration (mol/L)	Equivalent	Normality (N)
Hydrochloric acid	HCl	36.46	20%	1.10	6.0	1	6.0
			35%	1.17	11.2		11.2
Nitric acid	HNO_3	63.01	60%	1.37	13.0	1	13.0
			65%	1.39	14.3		14.3
			70%	1.41	15.7		15.7
Sulfate	H_2SO_4	98.08	100%	1.83	18.7	2	37.3
Phosphoric acid	H_3PO_4	98.00	85%	1.69	14.7	3	44.0
			90%	1.75	16.1		48.2
Acetate	CH_3COOH	60.05	100%	1.05	17.5	1	17.5
Perchloric acid	$HClO_4$	100.46	60%	1.54	9.2	1	9.2
			70%	1.67	11.6		11.6
Hydrogen peroxide water	H_2O_2	34.01	30%	1.11	9.8	-	
			35%	1.13	11.6		
Ammonia water	NH_3	17.03	25%	0.91	13.4	1	13.4
			28%	0.90	14.8		14.8

【Quick reference of concentration and unit】

● How to express concentration of solution

Expression	Commentary
Weight percent concentration	"g number" of solute in 100g solution. Expressed as w/w%, wt%, and % for density in many cases.
Volume percent concentration	"m number" of solute in 100m solution. Expressed as v/v% when mixture or solute is liquid.
Weight versus volume percent concentration	"g number of solute in 100m of solution. Expressed as w/v%.
Normality	Gram equivalent number of solute in 1L solution. Expressed as N for capacity analysis.
Volume specific concentration	Concentration indirectly expressed by the volume ratio of diluting the liquid reagent. It is used in JIS and others. Example: Sulfuric acid (1 + 2) → Sulfuric acid is shown diluted with 2 volumes of water.
Weight ratio concentration	Concentration indirectly expressed by weight ratio at which solid reagent is dissolved. It is used in JIS and others. Example: Sodium chloride (1 + 19) →Dissolved in 19 weight of water with respect to 1 of NaCl.
Molarity	Mol number of target substance (solute) in 1L of solution. Expressed as mol/ or M.

- Prefix representing multiple

Express bigness		Express smallness		
$100 = 10^2$	h (Hecto)	$1/100 = 10^{-2}$	c (Centi)	% (Percent)
$1000 = 10^3$	k (Kilo)	$1/1000 = 10^{-3}$	m (Milli)	‰ (Permili)
100万 $= 10^6$	M (Mega)	1/100万 $= 10^{-6}$	μ (Micro)	ppm
1 Billion $= 10^9$	G (Giga)	1/10Billion $= 10^{-9}$	n (Nano)	ppb
1 Trillion $= 10^{12}$	T (Tera)	1/1 Trillion $= 10^{-12}$	p (Pico)	ppt
1000 Trillion $= 10^{15}$	p (Peta)	1/1000 Trillion $= 10^{-15}$	f (Femto)	ppq

- ppm Conversion table

ppb	ppm	%	mg/g	mg/L
1,000	1	0.0001	0.001	1
10,000	10	0.001	0.01	10
100,000	100	0.01	0.1	100
1,000,000	1,000	0.1	1	1,000
10,000,000	10,000	1	10	10,000

References

Alderighi, L., Gans, P., Ienco, A., Peters, D., Sabatini, A., Vacca, A. (1999). "Hyperquad simulation and speciation (HySS): a utility program for the investigation of equilibria involving soluble and partially soluble species". ***Coordination Chemistry Reviews., 184 (1): 311–318.***

Arduengo, P.M. (2010) Sloppy technicians and the progress of science. ***Promega Connections***

http://promega.wordpress.com/2010/03/15/sloppy-technicians.

Brown, et al. (2008) . Chemistry:The Central Science. 11th ed. Upper Saddle River, New Jersey: Pearson/Prentice Hall,.

"Buffer Reference Center". *Sigma-Aldrich. Archived from the original on 2009-04-17. Retrieved 2009-04-17.*

Butler, J. N. (1998). *Ionic Equilibrium: Solubility and pH calculations. Wiley. pp. 133–136.* ISBN 978-0-471-58526-8.

Carmody, W. R. (1961). "Easily prepared wide range buffer series". *J. Chem. Educ.*, **38** (11): 559–560.

Chang, Raymond. (2003). General Chemistry:The Essential Concepts. 3rd ed. New York: Mcgraw Hill .

Good, N.E. *et al*. (1966) Hydrogen ion buffers for biological research. Biochemistry., 5 : 467–77.

Hulanicki, A. (1987). *Reactions of acids and bases in analytical chemistry. Translated by Masson, Mary R. Horwood.* ISBN 978-0-85312-330-9.

McIlvaine, T. C. (1921). "A buffer solution for colorimetric comparaison" (PDF). J. Biol. Chem. , 49 (1) : 183–186.. Archived (PDF) *from the original on 2015-02-26.*

Mendham, J. , Denny, R. C. , Barnes, J. D. , Thomas, M. (2000). "Appendix 5". Vogel's textbook of quantitative chemical analysis (5th ed.). Harlow: Pearson Education. ISBN 978-0-582-22628-9.

Petrucci, et al.(2007). General Chemistry: Principles & Modern Applications. 9th ed. Upper Saddle River, New Jersey: Pearson/Prentice Hall,.

Scorpio, R. (2000). *Fundamentals of Acids, Bases, Buffers & Their Application to* **Biochemical Systems**. ISBN 978-0-7872-7374-3.

Skoog, D. A., West, D.M., Holler, F. J., Crouch, S. R. (2014). *Fundamentals of Analytical Chemistry (9th ed.). Brooks/Cole. p. 226.* ISBN 978-0-495-55828-6

Stoll, V.S. and Blanchard, J.S. (1990) Buffers: Principles and practice. Meth. Enzymol. , 182:24–38.

Urbansky, E. T.and Schock, M. R. (2000). "Understanding, Deriving and Computing Buffer Capacity". **Journal of Chemical Education** *, 77 (12): 1640–1644.*

Contribution of Scientists in Endocrinological Research

Serial No.	Name of the Scientists	Time Period	Year of Discovery	Country of Origin (Birth Place)
	Adrenal Gland			
Adrenal Cortex				
1.	Edward Calvin Kendal	1886 - 1972	1950 (N.L.)	USA
2.	Tadeus Reichstein	1897- 1996	1950 (N.L.)	Poland
3.	Phillip Showalter Hench	1896-1965	1950 (N.L.)	USA
Adrenal Medulla				
1,	Sir Edward Albert Sharpey-Schafer	1850-1935		UK
2.	John Jacob Abel	1857-1938		USA
3.	Jokichi Takamine	1854-1922		JAPAN
Noradrenaline				

1.	Sir Bernard Katz	1911-2003	1970 (N.L.)	Germany
2.	Ulf von Euler	1905-1983	1970 (N.L.)	Sweden
3.	Julius Axelrod	1912-2004	1970 (N.L.)	USA
	Testis			
1.	Professor Enrico Sertoli	1842-1910	1865	Italy
2.	Franz von Leydig	1821-1908	1850	Germany
3	Butenandt , Adolf	1903-1995	1939	Germany
4.	Leopold Ruzica	1887-1976	1939	Croatia
	Ovary			
1.	Reiner de Graaf	1641-1673		Netherlands
	Thyroid Gland			
1.	Emil Theodor Kocher	1841-1917	1909 (N.L.)	Switzerland

		Parathyroid Gland			
	1.	James Bertram Collip	1892-1965		Canada
		Thymus Gland			
	1.	Professor Jacques Miller	19331- Alive		Australia
		Kidney			
	1.	Robert Adolph armand Tigerstedt	1853-1923		Finland
	2.	Harry Goldblatt	1891-1977		France
		Pancreas			
	1.	Derick Grant Banting	1891- 1941	1923 (N.L.)	Canada
	2.	John James Rickard Macleod	1876-1935	1923 (N.L.)	Scotland
		Liver			

1.	Karl Wilhelm von Kupffer	1829-1902	1876	Germany
	Pituitary			
Anterior Pituitary				
1.	Bernardo Alberto Housey	1887-1971	1947 (N.L.)	Argentina
2.	Carl ferdinando Cori	1896-1984	1947 (N.L.)	Czech Republic
3.	Gerty Theresa Cori, nee Radnitz	1896-1957	1947 (N.L.)	Czech Republic
4.	Roger Guillemin	1924- Alive	1977 (N.L.)	France
5.	Andrew V. Schally	1926-Alive	1977 (N.L.)	Poland
6.	Rosalyn Yallow	1921-2011	1977 (N.L.)	USA
Posterior Pituitary				
1.	Percy Theodore Herring	1872-1967	1908	UK

2.	Vincent du Vigneaud	1901-1978	1955 (N.L.)	USA

ASSOCIATWD FELLOW ENGAGED IN ENDOCRINOLOGICAL RESEARCH

1.	Charles Herbert Best/	1899-1978	Collaborated with Banting (NL)	Canada
2	James Bertram Collip	1892-1965	Played a central role in isolating Insulin and associated with Macleod (NL)	Canada
3.	Per Gustaf Bergman	1874 - 1955	Closely associated with Professor Robert A.A.Tigerstedt	Stockholm (Sweden)
4.	Solomon A. Berson	1918-1972	Solomon A. Berson helped Yalow(NL) to develop RIA	USA

REFERENCES

Agronskaia, A.V., Valentijn, J.A., van Driel ,L.F., Schneijdenberg, C.T.W.M., Humbel, B.M., van Bergen en Henegouwen, P.M.P., Verkleij, A.J., Koster, A.J., Gerritsen, H.C.(2008). Integrated fluorescence and transmission electron microscopy. J Struct Biol. , 164(2):183–189.

Aijaz, S., Clark, B.J., Williamson, K., van Heyningen ,V., Morrison, D., Fitzpatrick, D., Collin, R., Ragge, N., Christoforou, A., Brown, A., Hanson, I. (2004) . Absence of SIX6 mutations in microphthalmia, anophthalmia, and coloboma. Investigative ophthalmology & visual science. , 45 : 3871-3876.

Altman, L.G., Schneider, B.G., and Papermaster, D.S.(1984) . Rapid embedding of tissues in Lowicryl K4M for immunoelectron microscopy ., J. Histochem. Cytochem., 32 : 1217–1223 .

Ananthanarayanan ,V., Pins, M.R., Meyer, R.E., Gann, P.H.(2005) . Immunohistochemical assays in prostatic biopsies processed in Bouin's fixative. J Clin Pathol ., 58(3):322–324

Anderson, J. (2011) . An introduction to Routine and special staining. Retrieved on August 18, 2014 from
http://www.leicabiosystems.com/pathologyleaders/an-introduction-to-routine-and-special-staining.

Arnolds, W. J. (1978) . Oriented embedding of small objects in agar-paraffin, with reference marks for serial section reconstruction. Stain Technol., 53: 287–288 .

Aschoff, A., Fritz, N., and Ilert, M. (1982) . Axonal transport of fluorescent compounds in the brain and spinal cord of cat and rat, in Axonal Transport in Physiology and Pathology, Weiss, D.G. and Gorio, A., Eds., Springer, Berlin, 1982, p. 177.

Alturkistani, H.A., Tashkandi, F.M., Mohammedsaleh, Z.M.(2015) . Histological stains : a literature review and case study . Glob J Health Sci., 8:72-9. 10.5539/gjhs.v8n3p72.

Auinger, S. , Small, J.V. (2008). Correlated light and electron microscopy of the cytoskeleton . Methods Cell Biol., 88: 257–272.

Bachmann, L. and Salpeter, E.E. (1965) . Autoradiography with the electron microscope. A quantitative investigation, Lab. Invest., 14 : 1041–1051 .

Baker, J.R. (1958a) . Experiments on fixation , Unpublished observations, 1958a.

Baker, J.R. (1958b). Principles of Biological Microtechnique, 1st ed., Methuen & Co. Ltd., London .

Baker, F.J. , Silverstone, R.E. (1976). Introduction to Medical Laboratory Technology. 5th ed. Butterworth-Heinemann .

Bancroft, J.D. and Stevens, A. (1990) . Theory and Practice of Histological Techniques, Churchill Livingstone, Edinburgh .

Bancroft, J.D. and Layton, C. (2013) . The Hematoxylin and Eosin. In: Suvarna, S.K., Layton, C. and Bancroft, J.D., Eds., Theory & Practice of Histological Techniques, 7th Edition, Churchill Livingstone of El Sevier, Philadelphia, Ch. 10 and 11, 172-214.
https://doi.org/10.1016/B978-0-7020-4226-3.00010-X.

Beckman, W.C.J., Stumpf, W.E., and Sar, M. (1983). Localisation of steroid hormones and their receptors. A comparison of autoradiographic and immunocytochemical techniques, in Techniques in Imunocytochemistry, Bullock, G.R. and Petrusz, P., Eds., Academic Press, London.

Bennett, H.S., Wyrick, A.D., Lee, S.W., and McNeil, J.H. (1976) . Science and art in preparing tissues embedded in plastic for light microscopy, with special reference to glycol methacrylate, glass knives and simple stains, Stain Technol., 51: 71–97 .

Berry, C.L., Sosa-Melgarejo, J.A. , and Greenwald, S.E. (1993) . The relationship between wall tension, lamellar thickness and intercellular junctions in the fetal and adult aorta: its relevance to the pathology of dissecting aneurysm, J. Pathol., 169 : 15–20 .

Bibb, C.A., Pullinger, A.G., and Baldioceda, F. (1993) . Serial variation in histological character of articular soft tissue in young human adult temporomandibular joint condyles , Arch. Oral Biol., 38 : 343–352 .

Black , J. (2012.) . Microbiology : Principles and exploration. 8th ed. John Wiley Sons; p. 68.

Bradbury, S. and Bracegirdle, B. (1998) . Introduction to Light Microsocopy, Royal Microscopical Society Handbooks, Vol. 42, BIOS Scientific Publishers, Oxford .

Branchereau, P., Van Bockstaele, E.J., Chan, J., and Pickel, V.M.(1995). Ultrastructural characterization of neurons recorded intracellularly in vivo and injected with lucifer yellow: advantages of immunogold-silver vs. immunoperoxidase labeling, Microsc. Res. Tech., 30 : 427–436 .

Bancroft, J.D. , Stevens, A. (1995) . Theory and Practice of Histological Techniques. 4th Ed., Churchill-Livingstone, New York .

Bancroft, J.D., Gamble M. (2002). Theory and Practice of Histological Techniques. 5th ed. Philadelphia, PA: Churchill Livingstone Elsevier ; 63–108.

Baker, J.R. (1958) . Principles of Biological Microtechnique. John Wiley & Sons, Inc., New York .

Beach, T.G. , Tago, H. and Nagai, T. (1987) . "Perfusion-fixation of the Human Brain for Immunohistochemistry: Comparison with Immersion-Fixation," J. Neurosci Methods , 19(3) : 183-192 .

Bedran-Russo, A.K. , Pereira, P.N., Duarte, W.R. Drummond, J.L., Yamauchi , M. (2007). Application of crosslinkers to dentin collagen enhances the ultimate tensile strength. J Biomed Mater Res B Appl Biomater , 80(1) : 268–272 .

Beisker, W. , Dolbeare, F. , and Gray, J. W. (1987) . An improved immunocytochemical procedure for high-sensitivity detection of incorporated bromodeoxyuridine. Cytometry, 8 : 235-239.

Berestecky, John. (2008) . Microscopy : In Microbiology 140. Retrieved from http://www2.hawaii.edu/~johnb/micro/m140/syllabus/week/handouts/m140.2.4.html.

Berger, P., Berger, I., Schaffitzel, C., Tersar, K., Volkmer, B., & Suter, U. (2006). Multi-level regulation of myotubularin- related protein - 2 phosphatase activity by myotubularin related protein-13/set-binding factor-2. Hum Mol Genet . , 15 : 569–579.

Betterton, E.A., Hoffmann, M.R. (1988) . Henry's law constants of some environmentally important aldehydes. Environ. Sci . Technol. , 22(12) :

Blueford, J.R. (n.d.). Classification of microscopes. In Microscopes. Retrieved from http://www.msnucleus.org/membership/html/jh/biological/microscopes/lesson2/microscopes2c.html.

Bondonna, T.J. , Jacquet, Y. and Wolf, G. (1977). "Perfusion-Fixation Procedure for Immediate Histological Processing of Brain Tissue", Physiol. Behav. , 19(2) : 345-347.

Bozzola, J.J., Russell, L.D. (1992). Electron microscopy: principles and techniques for biologists. Boston: Jones and Bartlett .

Bracegirdle, B (1977) . The history of histology : A brief survey of sources. Hist Sci. , 77-101. doi:10.1177/007327537701500201

Bracegirdle B.(1977) . J. J. lister and the establishment of histology. Med Hist. , 21(2) : 187-191. doi:10.1017/S0025727300037716.

Cai, H., Caswell, J. L., Prescott, J. F. (March 2014). Nonculture Molecular Techniques for Diagnosis of Bacterial Disease in Animals: A Diagnostic Laboratory Perspective. Veterinary Pathology , 51(2):341–350.http://dx.doi.org/10.1177/0300985813511132 .

Calvo, J. And Boya, J. (1984) . Ultrastructure of the pineal gland in the adult rat J. Anat. , 138(3) : 405-409.

Cammermeyer, J. (1978) . "Is the Solitary Dark Neuron a Manifestation of Postmortem Trauma to the Brain Inadequately Fixed by Perfusion?" Histochemistry , 56 : 97-115 .

Carlsson, K., Danielsson, P.E., Lenz, R., Liljeborg, A., Majlof, L., and Aslund, N.(1985) . Three-dimensional microscopy using a confocal laser scanning microscope, Opt. Lett., 10 : 53–55,.

Carleton, H.M., Drury, R.A.B., Wallington, E.A.(1980) . Carleton's Histological Technique. 5th ed. New York, NY: Oxford University Press.

Carson, F.L. (1990) . Histopathology : A Self-Instructional Text, 2nd Ed., ASCP Press, Chicago, IL.

Carson, F.L. (1997) . Histotechnology . A Self-Instructional Text. 2nd Edition, American Society for Clinical Pathology Press, Chicago, 160.

Carson, F.L. , Edgar, L.C., Tatum, D.S.(2001). Board of Registry Study Guide: Histotechnology Examinations. 2nd ed. ASCP Press, Chicago, IL .

Carson, F.L. , Hladik Cappellano, C. (2014) . Histotechnology : A Self-Instructional Text. 4th ed. Chicago, IL: ASCP Press .

Carson, F.L. (2007) . Histotechnology. 2nd ed. ASCP Press , Chicago .

Carson, F. L. , and Christa, H. (2009) . Histotechnology : A Self Instructional Text. 3rd ed. Chicago, Ill.: American Society of Clinical Pathologists,. 112 .

Carson, F.L. , Hladik, C. (2009) . Troubleshooting the H&E stain. In: Histotechnology a self-instructional text. 3rd ed. Chicago: American Society for Clinical Pathology Press; p. 118–122 .

Carson, F.L., Hladik , C. C. (2014) . Histotechnology : A Self-Instructional Text. 4th ed. Chicago, IL: ASCP Press .

Chan, J.K.C. (2014) . The wonderful colors of the hematoxylin-eosin stain in diagnostic surgical pathology. Int J Surg Pathol. , 22(1) : 12–32.

Chang, Y.T., Loew, G.H.(1994) . Reaction mechanisms of formaldehyde with endocyclic imino groups of nucleic acid bases. J Am Chem Soc. , 116(8) : 3548–3555 .

Chew, N.G., Cullis, A.G. (1987). The preparation of transmission electron microscope specimens from compound semiconductors by ion milling, Ultramicroscopy, 23(2) : 175-198.

Chiono, V. , Pulieri, E. , Vozzi , G. , Ciardelli , G. , Ahluwalia, A ., Giusti, P. (2008). Genipin-crosslinked chitosan/gelatin blends for biomedical applications. J Mater Sci Mater Med . , 19(2) : 889–898

Cinar, O., Semiz, O., & Can, A. (2006). A microscopic survey on the efficiency of well-known routine chemical fixatives on cryosections. Acta.Histochem. , 108 (6) : 487-96.

Clayden , E.C. (1971) . Practical section cutting and staining. Edinburgh: Churchill Livingstone .

Clermont, Y. , Oko, R., Hermo, L. (1993). Cell biology of mammalian spermiogenesis. In: Desjardin C, Ewing LL, editors. Cell and molecular biology of the testis. New York: Oxford University Press. pp. 332– 376.

Clermont, Y. (1991) . Four decades of research on the biology of the male reproductive system : A few landmarks. Ann NY Acad Sci . , 637 : 17– 25.

Clermont, Y. , Leblond, C. P . (1955) . Spermiogenesis of man, monkey, ram and other mammals as shown by the periodic acid-Schiff technique. Am J Anat., 96 : 229 – 253.

Clermont, Y., Rambourg, A. (1978) . Evolution of the endoplasmic reticulum during rat spermiogenesis. Am J Anat. , 151 : 191–211.

Clermont , Y. , Einberg , E. , Leblond, C.P., Wagner, S. (1955) . The perforatorium; an extension of the nuclear membrane of the rat spermatozoon. Anat Rec., 121 : 1–12 .

Cogan JD, Wu W, Phillips JA, 3rd, Arnhold IJ, Agapito A, Fofanova OV, Osorio MG, Bircan I, Moreno A, Mendonca BB (1998) . The PROP1 2-base pair 214 deletion is a common cause of combined pituitary hormone deficiency. J Clin Endocrinol Metab. , 83:3346-3349

Colombelli, J., Tangemo, C., Haselman, U., Antony, C., Stelzer, E. H., Pepperkok, R., Emmanuel G Reynaud, E.G. (2008). A correlative light and electron microscopy method based on laser micropatterning and etching. Methods Mol. Biol. , 457 : 203–213. doi: 10.1007/978-1-59745-261-8_15.

Coons, A.H., Creech, H.J. and Jones, R.N. (1941) Immunological Properties of an Antibody Containing a Fluorescent Group. Experimental Biology and Medicine, 47 : 200-202. https://doi.org/10.3181/00379727-47-13084p.

Coons, A. H., Creech, H. J., Jones, R. N. & Berliner, G. (1942) . The demonstration of pneumococcal antigen in tissues by the use of fluorescent antibody. J. Immunology , 45 : 159-170 .

Coons, A.H. and Kaplan, M.H. (1950). Localization of antigen in tissue cells, J. Exp. Med., 91: 1–13,.

Coons, A.H., Leduce, E.H., and Connolly, J.M.(1955) . Studies on antibody production. I. A method for the histochemical demonstration of specific antibody and its application to a study of the hyperimmune rabbit, J. Exp. Med., 102 : 49–60 .

Costa, C. A. X. , Brito, K. N. O. , Gomes, M. A., Caliari, M. V. (2010) . Histopathological and immunohistochemical study of the hepatic lesions experimentally induced by Entamoeba dispar ., European Journal of Histochemistry, 54 : 170-174.

Cowen, T., Haven, A. J., and Burnstock, G. (1985) . Pontamine sky blue: a counterstain for background autofluorescence in fluorescence and immunofluorescence histochemistry. Histochemistry , 82 : 205-208 .

Cragg, B. (1980) . Preservation of extracellular space during fixation of the brain for electron microscopy. Tissue Cell, 12 : 63 - 72.

Creasy, D.M., and Foster, P.M.D. (2002). Male reproductive system, in Handbook of toxicologic pathology (Haschek, W.M., Rousseaux, C.G., and Wallig, M.A., eds), Vol. 2. Academic Press, San Diego New York Boston, pp 785–846.

Culling, C.F.A., Allison, R.T., and Barr, W.T. (1985) . Cellular Pathology Technique, 4th ed., London, Butterworths, London, 32.

Culling, C.F.A. (1985) . A Handbook of Histopathological and Histochemical Techniques. 4th ed. London: Butterworth Publication ; 27–77.

Cummings, J.F. and Petras, J.M. (1977) . The Origin of Spinocerebellar Pathways 1. The Nucleus Cervicalis Centralis of the Cranial - Cervical Spinal Cord. J. Comp. Neurt., 173: 655 - 692 .

Darcy , K.J., Staras, K. , Collinson, L.M., Goda, Y. (2006) . Constitutive sharing of recycling synaptic vesicles between presynaptic boutons. Nat Neurosci., 9 : 315–321.

Darcy, K,J., Staras, K. , Collinson, L.M ., Goda, Y. (2006). An ultrastructural readout of fluorescence recovery after photobleaching using correlative light and electron microscopy. Nat Protoc., 1: 988–994.

Dasen, J.S., O'Connell, S.M. , Flynn, S.E., Treier, M., Gleiberman, A.S., Szeto, D.P., Hooshmand, F., Aggarwal ,A.K., Rosenfeld, M.G.(1999) . Reciprocal interactions of Pit1 and GATA2 mediate signaling gradient-induced determination of pituitary cell types. Cell, 97 : 587-598.

Davis, S.W. , Castinetti, F., Carvalho, L.R., Ellsworth, B . S., Po.tok, M.A., Lyons , R.H., Brinkmeier, M.L., Raetzman, L.T., Carninci, P., Mortensen, A.H., Hayashizaki, Y., Arnhold, I.J., Mendonca, B.B., Brue, T., Camper ,S.A.(2010) . Molecular mechanisms of pituitary organogenesis: In search of novel regulatory genes. Mol Cell Endocrinol., 323 : 4-19.

Deladoey, J. , Fluck, C., Buyukgebiz, A., Kuhlmann, B.V., Eble, A., Hindmarsh, P.C., Wu, W. , Mullis, P.E.(1999). "Hot spot" in the PROP1 gene responsible for combined pituitary hormone deficiency. J Clin Endocrinol Metab., 84 : 1645-1650 .

Dobrin, P.B. (1996). Effect of histologic preparation on the cross-sectional area of arterial rings, J. Surg. Res., 61: 413–415 .

Dode, C. , Levilliers, J., Dupont, J.M. , De Paepe, A. , Le Du, N., Soussi-Yanicostas, N. , Coimbra, R.S. , Delmaghani, S ., Compain-Nouaille , S ., Baverel, F ., Pecheux , C. , Le Tessie, D. , Cruaud, C. , Delpech, M ., Speleman, F. , Vermeulen, S . , Amalfitano, A. , Bachelot ,Y. , Bouchard, P. , Cabrol, S ., Carel ,J.C. , Delemarre-van de Waal, H. , Goulet-Salmon, B. , Kottler, M.L.,   .Richard, O., Sanchez-Franco, F., Saura, R. , Young, J. , Petit, C. , Hardelin, J.P. (2003) . Loss-of-function mutations in FGFR1 cause autosomal dominant Kallmann syndrome. Nature genetics , 33 : 463-465.

Donath, K. (1985) . The diagnostic value of the new method for the study of undecalcified bones and teeth with attached soft tissue (Sage-Schliff (sawing and grinding) technique), Pathol. Res. Pract., 179 : 631–633 .

Doniach, I. and Pelc, S.R., Autoradiographic technique, Br. J. Radiogr., 23, 184–192, 1950.

Douglas K. R.. and Tyla, S.F. (2010) . Transmission electron microscopy of cartilage and bone. Methods in Cell Biology, 96 : 443-73 .

Dove ,.S.K., Cooke, .F.T. , Douglas, M.R. , Sayers, L.G., Parker, P.J., et al. (1997) . Osmotic stress activates phosphatidylinositol-3,5-bisphosphate synthesis. Nature , 390 : 187–192.

Drury, R.A.B. and Wallington, E.A. (1980). Carleton's Histological Technique, 5th ed., Oxford University Press, Oxford, 1980.

Durmaz, B . , Cogulu, O., Dizdarer, C ., Stobbe, H. , Pfaeffle, R. , Ozkinay, F.(2011) A novel homozygous HESX1 mutation causes panhypopituitarism without midline defects and optic nerve anomalies. Journal of pediatric endocrinology & metabolism : JPEM , 24 : 779-782.'

Dyba, M. and Hell, S.W. (2002). Focal spots of size lambda/23 open up far-field fluorescence microscopy at 33 nm axial resolution, Phys. Rev. Lett., 88 : 163901-1–163901- 4.

Drury, R.A.B., Wallington, E.A . (1980). Carleton's histological technique . 5th ed. New York: Churchill Livingstone.

Edington, J.W. (1974). Practical Electron Microscopy in Materials Science, Vols. 1-5, 1974, Philips, Eindhoven.

Egger, M.D. and Petran, M.(1967). New reflected-light microscope for viewing unstained brain and ganglion cells. Science, 157 : 305–307.

Ellis, R. C. (1994). The microtome function and design , in Laboratory histopathology, a complete reference (Woods, A.E., and Ellis, R.C., eds), Churchill Livingstone, New York, Vol. 1, pp 4.4-1/4.4-23.

Eltoum, I.E., Freenburgh, J. , Myers, R.B. , Grizzle, W.E.(2001). Introduction to the theory and practice of fixation of tissues. J Histotechnol ,24(3) : 173–190.

Eltoum, I. , Fredenburgh ,J., Grizzle, W.E . (2001). Advanced concepts in fixation : 1. Effects of fixation on immunohistochemistry, reversibility of fixation and recovery of proteins, nucleic acids, and other molecules from fixed and processed tissues. 2. Developmental methods of fixation. J Histotechnol, 24(3) : 201–210.

Falardeau, J. , Chung, W.C.J., Beenken , A. , Raivio, T. Plummer, L. , Sidis, Y. , Jacobson-Dickman, E.E. , Eliseenkova, A.V. , Ma J., Dwyer, A. , Quinton, R. , Na ,S., Hall, J.E., Huot ,C., Alois, N., Pearce, S.H., Cole, L.W., Hughes, V., Mohammadi, M., Tsai, P. , Pitteloud, N. (2008). Decreased FGF8 signaling causes deficiency of gonadotropin-releasing hormone in humans and mice., J. Clin. Invest. ,118 : 2822-2831.

Fisher Scientific. MSDS :Glyoxal. 2008; . http://fscimage.fishersci.com/msds/01960.htm; November 22, 2011.

Fox, C.H. , Johnson, F.B. , Whiting, J. , Roller, P.P. (1985). Formaldehyde fixation. J Histochem Cytochem. , 33(8) : 845–853

Freida ,L . , Carson, C.H.C.(2009) . (Histotechnology: A Self Instructional Text. 3rd ed. American Society for Clinical Pathology Press, Hong Kong .

French, D., Edsall, J.T.(1945). The reactions of formaldehyde with amino acids and proteins. Adv Pro Cherlz , 2:277–335 .

Fritz, M., Rinaldi, G. (2008) . Blood pressure measurement with the tail-cuff method in Wistar and spontaneously hypertensive rats: Influence of adrenergic- and nitric oxide-mediated vasomotion. J. Pharmacol. Toxicol. Methods. , 58 : 215-221.

Gage, G. J. , Kipke, D. R. , Shain, W. (2012) . Whole Animal Perfusion Fixation for Rodents. J. Vis. Exp., (65): e3564, doi:10.3791/3564. **(Revised: February 28, 2019).**

Gaietta ,G.M., Giepmans, B.N., Deerinck, T.J., Smith, W.B. , Ngan, L., Llopes, J., Adams, S.R., Tsien, R.Y., Ellisman, M.H. (2006). Golgi twins in late mitosis revealed by genetically encoded tags for live cell imaging and correlated electron microscopy. Proc Natl Acad Sci U S A, 103 : 17777–17782.

Gamble M. The hematoxylins and eosin. In: Bancroft JD, Gamble M, editors. Theory and practice of histological techniques. 6th ed. London (UK): Churchill Livingston/Elsevier Inc; 2008. p. 121–134.

Gaston-Massuet, C., Andoniadou, C.L., Signore, M., Sajedi, E., Bird, S., Turner, J.M., Martinez-Barbera, J.P. (2008). Genetic interaction between the homeobox transcription factors HESX1 and SIX3 is required for normal pituitary development. Developmental biology, 324 : 322-333.

Gaston-Massuet, C., Andoniadou, C.L. , Signore, M., Jayakody, S.A., Charolidi, N. , Kyeyune, R., Vernay, B., Jacques, T.S., Taketo, M.M., Le Tissier, P., Dattani, M.T., Martinez-Barbera, J.P. (2011) . Increased Wingless (Wnt) signaling in pituitary progenitor/stem cells gives rise to pituitary tumors in mice and humans. Proc Natl Acad Sci U S A, 108 : 11482-11487.

Gareth ,T. and Michael, J.(1979). Goringe, Transmission Electron Microscopy of Materials, John Wiley & Sons, New York.

Gertz, S.D., Rennels, M.C. , Forbes, M .S. and Nelson, E. (1975). "Preparation of Vascular Endothelium for Scanning Electron Microscopy: A Comparison of the Effects of Perfusion and Immersion Fixation," J . Microsc. , 105(3) : 309-313 .

Glauert, A.M., Lewis, P.R. (1998) . Biological Specimen Preparation for Transmission Electron Microscopy. Princeton University Press , Princeton , NJ..

Godwin, A.(2011) . Histochemical uses of haematoxylin - a review. [Retrieved August 18, 2014]. From www.arpapress.com .

Gormley, B., and Ellis, R.C. (1994). Resin embedding for light microscopy, in Laboratory histopathology, a complete reference (Woods, A.E., and Ellis, R.C., eds), Churchill Livingstone, New York, Vol. 1, pp 4.3-1/4.3-13.

Grabenbauer, M. , Geerts, W.J., Fernadez-Rodriguez, J. , Hoenger, A., Koster, A.J., Nilsson, T. (2005) . Correlative microscopy and electron tomography of GFP through photooxidation. Nat Methods , 2: 857–862.

Griffiths, G. , McDowall, A., Back, R., Dubochet, J. (1984). On the preparation of cryosections for immunocytochemistry., J Ultrastruct Res., 89 : 65–78.

Gruska M, Medalia O, Baumeister W, Leis A (2008) Electron tomography of vitreous sections from cultured mammalian cells. J Struct Biol. , 161: 384–392.

Guidelines for Hematoxylin & Eosin Staining. National Society for Histotechnology. Published by NSH Office, Bowie, MD. 2001.

Ham, A.W., Cormack, D.H. (1987) . Ham's Histology. 9th ed. Philadelphia, PA: Lippincott.

Hansen, J.T. (2002) . Essential Anatomy Dissector Following Grant's Method. 2nd ed. Philadelphia, PA: Lippincott Williams & Wilkins .

Hansen, J.T.(2002) . Essential Anatomy Dissector Following Grant's Method. 2nd ed.
Philadelphia, PA: Lippincott Williams & Wilkins .
Harke, H.P., Höffler, J. (1984) . Übergang antimikrobieller Wirkstoffe von der Fläche in die Luft. Hyg Med. , 9 : 259–260.

Hayat ,M.A.(1984). Fixation for Electron Microscopy. Academic Press , New York, NY.

Hayat ,M.A. (1981) . Principles and Techniques of Electron Microscopy. Biological Applications. 2nd ed, Vol. 1: University Park Press, Baltimore, MD.

Harris, T. J, McCormick, F. (2010) . The molecular pathology of cancer. Nat Rev Clin Oncol. , 7(5):251–265.
http://dx.doi.org/10.1038/nrclinonc.2010.41 . [PubMed] [Google Scholar]

Hassell, J. , Hand, A.R. (1974). Tissue fixation with diimidoesters as an alternative to aldehydes. I. Comparison of cross-linking and ultrastructure obtained with dimethylsuberimidate and glutaraldehyde. J Histochem Cytochem. , 22(4): 229-239.

Hayat, M.A. (1993) . Stains and Cytochemical Methods. Plenum Press , New York, NY; London, UK.

Hayat, M.A. (2000). Principles and Techniques of Electron Microscopy, Biological Applications, fourth ed., Cambridge University Press, Cambridge .

Heindel, J.J., and Chapin, R.E. (1993). Female reproductive toxicology, in Methods in reproductive toxicology (Heindel, J.J., and Chapin, R.E., eds), Vol. 3B, Academic Press, Orlando.

Hess ,M.W., Muller, M. , Debbage, P.L . , Vetterlein, M ., Pavelka, M. (2000) . Cryopreparation provides new insight into the effects of brefeldin A on the structure of the HepG2 Golgi apparatus. J Struct Biol . , 130: 63–7.

Hohenberg, H. , Mannweiler, K. , Muller, M. (1994). High-pressure freezing of cell suspensions in cellulose capillary tubes. J Microsc., 175 : 34–43.

Hopwood, D. (1967). Some aspects of fixation with glutaraldehyde. A biochemical and histochemical comparison of the effects of formaldehyde and glutaraldehyde fixation on various enzymes and glycogen, with a note on penetration of glutaraldehyde into liver. J Anat . , 101(Pt 1) : 83–92 .

Hopwood, D. (1969) . Fixatives and fixation: a review. Histochem J . , 1(4) : 323–360

Hopwood, D . (1973) . Fixation with mercury salts. Acta Histochem Supp ., 13(0) : 107–118.

Hopwood, D.(1985). Cell and tissue fixation, 1972–1982. Histochern J . , 17(4) : 389–442 .

Hopwood, D. , Milne, G., Penston, J. (1990) . A comparison of microwaves and heat alone in the preparation of tissue for electron microscopy. Histochem J . , 22(6-7) : 358–364

Hopwood, D. (1996) . Fixation and fixatives. In Bancroft, J. and Stevens, A. eds. Theory and practice of histological techniques. , Churchill Livingstone , New York .

Hornickel, I. , Kacza , J. , Schnapper , A. , Beyerbach , M. , Schoennagel , B. , Seeger, J. , Meyer, W. (2011) . Demonstration of substances of innate immunity in the esophagus epithelium of domesticated mammals. Part I—methods and comparative fixation evaluation. Acta Histochem., 113(2) : 175–188 .

Hussein, I.H., Raad, M. (2015) . Once Upon a Microscopic Slide: The Story of Histology. J Cytol Histol., 6(6) : 1-4. doi:10.4172/2157-7099.1000377.

Horvath , E. , Kovacs, K. (2002). Folliculo-stellate cells of the human pituitary: a type of adult stem cell? Ultrastructural pathology , 26 : 219-228

Ikeda, K., Nara, Y., Yamorii, Y. (1991) . Indirect systolic and mean blood pressure determination by anew tail cuff method in spontaneously hypertensive rats . Laboratory Animals., **25** : 26-29.

Ingraham, H.A., Lala, D.S., Ikeda, Y., Luo, X., Shen, W.H., Nachtigal, M.W., Abbud, R., Nilson, J.H., Parker, K.L. (1994) . The nuclear receptor steroidogenic factor 1 acts at multiple levels of the reproductive axis. Genes & development , 8 : 2302-2312.

Iyiola, S. and Avwioro, O. G. (2011) . Alum haematoxylin stain for the demonstration of nuclear and extra nuclear substances. Journal of Pharmacy and Clinical Sciences, 1: 20-23.

Jackson, P. , Blythe, D. (2013) . Theory Practice of histological techniques. In SK. Suvarna , C. Layton , JD. Bancroft (Eds. 7th ed. Ch. 18. Philadelphia: Churchill Livingstone of El Sevier; Immunohistochemical techniques ; pp. 386–431. http://dx.doi.org/10.1016/b978-0-7020-4226-3.00018-4 .

Jacobowitz, D. M. (1974) . Removal of discrete fresh regions of rat brain. Brain Res., **80** :111-115.

Jimenez, N., Humbel, B.M., van Donselaar, E., Verkleij, A.J., Burger, K.N. (2006). Aclar discs: a versatile substrate for routine high-pressure freezing of mammalian cell monolayers. J Microsc., 221 : 216–223.

John, C.D., Theogaraj, E. , Christian, H.C., Morris, J.F., Smith, S.F., Buckingham, J.C. (2006). Time-specific effects of perinatal glucocorticoid treatment on anterior pituitary morphology, annexin 1 expression and adrenocorticotrophic hormone secretion in the adult female rat. J Neuroendocrinol . , 18 : 949-959

Johnson, W.D. , Lang, C.M. and Johnson, M.T. (1978) . Fixatives and Methods of Fixation in Selected Tissues of the Laboratory Rat , Clinical Toxicology, 12(5) : 583-600 .

Jonkers, B.W., Sterk , J.C. , & Wouterlood, F.G. (1984) . Transcardial perfusion fixation of the CNS by means of a compressed-air-driven device. Journal of Neurosci. Meth. , 12 (2) : 141-149 .

Jung-Hwa, T. ao-C. heng, Gallant, J., Brightman, P. E., Dosemeci, M. W., A,, Reese, T. S. (2007). Structural changes at the synapse after delayed perfusion fixation in different regions of the mouse brain. J. Comp. Neurol. , 501 : 731-740

Kalimo, H. , Rehncrona, S., Soderfeldt, B. , Olsson, Y. and Siesjo, B.K. (1981) . "Brain Lactic Acidosis and Ischemic Cell Damage : 2. Histopathology, J. of Cerebral Blood Flow and Metabolism ., 1 : 313- 327

Kasukurthi, R., Brenner, M. J., Morre, A. M., Moradzadeh, A., Wilson, Z. R., Santosa, K. B., Mackinnon, S. E., Hunter, D. A. (2009). Transcardial perfusion versus immersion fixation for assessment of peripheral nerve regeneration. J. Neurosci. Meth. , 184 : 303-309 .

Kelberman , D. , Dattani, M.T. (2009). Role of transcription factors in midline central nervous system and pituitary defects. Endocrine development ., 14: 67-82.

Kelberman, D. , Rizzoti, K. , Lovell-Badge, R. , Robinson, I.C., Dattani, M.T. (2009) Genetic regulation of pituitary gland development in human and mouse. Endocr Rev., 30 : 790-829.

Kelberman, D. , de Castro, S.C., Huang, S., Crolla, J.A., Palmer, R., Gregory, J.W., Taylor, D., Cavallo ,L. , Faienza, M.F., Fischetto, R., Achermannm, J.C., Martinez-Barbera ,J.P., Rizzoti, K., Lovell-Badge, R., Robinson, I.C., Gerrelli, D., Dattani, M.T. (2008) . SOX2 plays a critical role in the pituitary, forebrain, and eye during human embryonic development . J Clin Endocrinol Metab ., 93 :1865 -1873

Kelberman, D., Rizzoti, K., Avilion, A., Bitner-Glindzicz ,M. , Cianfarani, S., Collins, J., Chong ,W.K., Kirk, J.M., Achermann ,J.C., Ross, R., Carmignac, D., Lovell-Badge ,R., Robinson ,I.C., Dattani, M.T.(2006). Mutations within Sox2/SOX2 are associated with abnormalities in the hypothalamo-pituitary-gonadal axis in mice and humans. J Clin Invest . , 116 : 2442-2455.

Kiernan, J.A. (2008) . Histological and Histochemical Methods : Theory and Practice . 4 th ed, Scion, Bloxham, UK .

Kioussi ,C., Briata, P., Baek, S.H., Rose, D.W., Hamblet, N.S., Herman, T., Ohgi, K.A., Lin, C., Gleiberman, A., Wang, J., Brault, V., Ruiz-

Lozano, P., Nguyen, H.D., Kemler, R., Glass ,C.K., Wynshaw-Boris, A., Rosenfeld, M.G.(2002). Identification of a Wnt/Dvl/beta-Catenin --> Pitx2 pathway mediating cell-type-specific proliferation during development. Cell , 111: 673 - 685.

Kita, A., Imayoshi, I., Hojo, M., Kitagawa, M., Kokubu, H., Ohsawa, R., Ohtsuka, T., Kageyama, R. , Hashimoto, N. (2007). Hes1 and Hes5 control the progenitor pool, intermediate lobe specification, and posterior lobe formation in the pituitary development. Mol Endocrinol ., 21:1458-1466.

Kittel, B. , Ruehl-Fehlert, C. , Morawietz, G. , Klapwijk, J. , Elwell, M.R. , Lenz, B. , O'Sullivan, M.G. , Roth, D.R. , and Wadsworth, P.F. (2004). Revised guides for organ sampling and trimming in rats and mice – Part 2. Exp. Toxic. Pathol. , 55:413–431.

Kremer, J.R., Mastronarde, D.N., McIntosh, J.R. (1996). Computer visualization of three-dimensional image data using IMOD. J Struct Biol., 116 : 71–76.

Lamberts, R. & Goldsmith, P.C. (1986) . Fixation, fine structure, and immunostaining for neuropeptides: perfusion versus immersion of the neuroendocrine hypothalamus. J. Histochem. Cytochem. , 34 : 389-398.

Lanning, L.L., Creasy, D.M., Chapin, R.E., Mann, P.C., Barlow, N.J., Regan, K.S., and Goodman, D.G. (2002). Recommended approaches for the evaluation of testicular and epididymal toxicity. Toxicol. Pathol. , 30 : 507–520.

Laporte, J., Hu, L.J., Kretz, C., Mandel, J.L., Kioschis, P., Coy, J.F., Klauck, S.M., Poustka, A. and Dahl, N. (1996) . A gene mutated in X-linked myotubular myopathy defines a new putative tyrosine phosphatase family conserved in yeast. Nature Genet., 13 : 175–182.

Larson, K., Ho, H.H., Anumolu, P.L., Chen, T.M. (2011) . Hematoxylin and eosin tissue stain in Mohs micrographic surgery: a review. Dermatol Surg. , 37(8) : 1089 - 99.

Latendresse, J.R., Warbrittion, A.R., Jonassen, H., and Creasy, D.M. (2002). Fixation of testes and eyes using a modified Davidson's fluid :

Comparison with Bouin's fluid and conventional Davidson's fluid. Toxicol. Pathol., 30: 524 – 533.

LeBlond, C.P., Clermont, Y. (1952) . Definition of the stages of the cycle of the seminiferous epithelium in the rat. Ann NY Acad Sci., 55:548 –573.

Lee, E. , Marcucci , M. , Daniell , L. , Pypaert , M., Weisz , O.A., Ochoa , G.C., Farsad , K. , Wenk , M.R. , De Camilli , P. (2002) . Amphiphysin 2 (Bin1) and T-tubule biogenesis in muscle. Science , 297 : 1193-1196.

Leica Microsystems. Instruction Manual Leica RM2235 V1.3 Nussloch: Leica Microsystems, 2008.

Leica, Microsystems. Material Safety Data Sheet: 10% Millonig's Buffered Formalin. 2007;
http://www.leicamicrosystems.com/index.php?id=1504&tx_leicaproducts_ pi1[showUid]=3299&tx_leicaproducts_pi1
[tab]=downloads&cHash=49baf1391ce5bcd25cd31e224782b369
27/10/2011 .

Leong, A.S.-Y. (1994). Fixation and fixatives, in Laboratory histopathology, a complete reference (In Woods, A.E., and Ellis, R.C., eds), Churchill Livingstone, New York, Vol. 1, pp 4.1-1/4.2-26.

Lester, S.C. (2010). Manual of Surgical Pathology. 3rd ed. Elsevier , New York , NY.

Lillie, R.D. , Fullmer, H.M. (1976) . Histopathologic Technique and Practical Histochemistry. 4th ed. New York, NY: McGraw-Hill .

Lillie, R.D. , Pizzolato, P. , Donaldson, P.T. (1976) . Nuclear stains with soluble metachrome mordant lake dyes. The effect of chemical endgroup blocking reactions and the artificial introduction of acid groups into tissues. Histochemistry, 49 : 23–35.

Luft , J.H. (1959). The use of acrolein as a fixative for light and electron microscopy. Anat Rec., 133 : 305

Luna, L.G.(1992) . Histopathologic Methods and Color Atlas of Special Stains and Tissue Artifacts. Gaithersburg, MD : American Histolabs .

Llewellyn, B.D .(2009). Nuclear staining with alum-hematoxylin. Biotech. Histochem. , 84 : 159–177.

Lott, R. , Tunnicliffe, J., Sheppard E, Santiago,J., Hladik,C., Nasim,M., Zeitner,K., Haas,T., Kohl,S., Lankarani, S.M. (2018). Practical guide to specimen handling in surgical pathology . CAP/NSH., revised .

Lowe , J. (1996). Techniques in neuropathology. In Bancroft JD and Stevens A eds. *Theory and practice of histological techniques*. New York: Churchill Livingstone, 373.

Lučić ,V., Kossel, A. H., Yang ,T., Bonhoeffer, T., Baumeister, W., and Sartori, A. (2007). Multiscale imaging of neurons grown in culture: from light microscopy to cryo-electron tomography. J. Struct. Biol. ,160:146-156.

Luna, Lee G.(1992) . Histopathologic Methods and Color Atlas of Special Stains and Tissue Artifacts. Gaitheresburg, MD: American Histolabs, 81-92.

Lyon, H. O., Horobin, R. W. (2010). Standardization and Standards for Dyes and Stains Used in Biology and Medicine. . [Retrieved August 18, 2014 from].http://www.dako.com/index/knowledgecenter/kc_publications/kc_pu blications_connection/kc_publications_connection14.htm/28829_2010_co nn14_std_dyes_stains_in_biology_lyon_and_horobin.pdf .

Machinis, K., Pantel, J., Netchine, I., Leger,J. , Camand, O.J., Sobrier, M.L., Dastot-Le Moal, F., Duquesnoy, P., Abitbol, M., Czernichow, P., Amselem ,S. (2001). Syndromic short stature in patients with a germline mutation in the LIM homeobox LHX4. American journal of human genetics, 69 : 961-968.

MacKenzie, S. A., Roher, N. , Boltana, S., Goetz, F. W. (2010) . Peptidoglycan, not endotoxin, is the key mediator of cytokine gene expression induced in rainbow trout macrophages by crude LPS. Mol Immunol. , 47:1450–1457.
http://dx.doi.org/10.1016/j.molimm.2010.02.009 . [PubMed] [Google Scholar]

Mascorro, J.A. and Bozzola, J.J. (2007). Processing biological tissues for ultrastructural study. In: Electron Microscopy. Methods and Protocols. Methods in Molecular Biology. Ed. John Kuo. Human Press.

Mastronarde, D.N. (1997). Dual-axis tomography: an approach with alignment methods that preserve resolution. J Struct Biol., 120 : 343–352.

Mayor, H.D., Jordan, L.E.(1963). Acrolein—a fine structure fixative for viral cytochemistry. J Cell Biol., 18(1) : 207–213.

McCabe , M.J. , Gaston-Massuet, C. , Tziaferi, V. , Gregory, L.C., Alatzoglou, K.S., Signore ,M., Puelles, E., Gerrelli, D., Farooqi, I.S., Raza, J., Walker, J., Kavanaugh, S.I., Tsai, P.S., Pitteloud, N., Martinez-Barbera, J.P. , Dattani, M.T.(2011). Novel FGF8 mutations associated with recessive holoprosencephaly, craniofacial defects, and hypothalamo-pituitary dysfunction. J Clin Endocrinol Metab., 96 : E1709-1718.

McGavin, M.D. (1991) Procedures for morphological studies of skeletal muscle, rat, mouse, and hamster, in Cardiovascular and musculoskeletal systems, Monographs on pathology of laboratory animals (Jones, T.C., Mohr U., and Hunt, R.D., eds), Springer, New York, pp 101–108.

McGhee, J.D. , von Hippel, P.H. (1975). Formaldehyde as a probe of DNA structure. I. Reaction with exocyclic amino groups of DNA bases. Biochemistry , 14(6) : 1281–1296

McGhee, J.D., von Hippel, P.H.(1975). Formaldehyde as a probe of DNA structure. II. Reaction with endocyclic imino groups of DNA bases. Biochemistry , 14(6):1297–1303.

McLennan, K. , Jeske, Y., Cotterill, A., Cowley, D. , Penfold, J. , Jones ,T., Howard ,N. , Thomsett, M., Choong, C.(2003) . Combined pituitary hormone deficiency in Australian children: clinical and genetic correlates. Clin Endocrinol. (Oxf) , 58:785-794.

McLeod, C.G. and Wall, H.G. (1987). "Pathology of Experimental Nerve Agent Poisoning." In: Neurobiology of Acetylcholine, edited by Nae J. Dun 'and Robert Perlman. Plenum Publishing Corp, pp. 427- 435 .

Medawar, P. B. (1941) . The rate of penetration of fixatives. J. Royal. Micros. Soc., 61: 46-57.

Meisslitzer-Ruppitsch, C., Rohrl, C., Neumuller, J., Pavelka, M., Ellinger, A. (2009). Photooxidation technology for correlated light and electron microscopy. J Microsc . , 235: 322–335.

Mironov, A.A., Polishchuk, R.S., Luini, A . (2000) . Visualizing membrane traffic in vivo by combined video fluorescence and 3D electron microscopy. Trends Cell Biol., 10: 349–353.

Mironov, A.A., Beznoussenko, G.V. (2009). Correlative microscopy : a potent tool for the study of rare or unique cellular and tissue events. J Microsc., 235 : 308–321.

Moolenbeek, C., and Ruitenberg, E.J. (1981). The "Swiss roll": a simple technique for histological studies of the rodent intestine. Lab. Anim. ,15: 57–59.

Monaghan, P. , Perusinghe, N. , Muller, M. (1998). High-pressure freezing for immunocytochemistry. J Microsc . , 192 : 248–258 .

Mongiu, A.K., Weitzke, E.L., Chaga, O.Y., Borisy, G.G. (2007). Kinetic-structural analysis of neuronal growth cone veil motility. J Cell Sci ., 120 : 1113–1125.

Morawietz, G., Ruehl-Fehlert, C., Kittel, B., Bube, A., Keane, K., Halm, S., Heuser, A., and Hellman, J. (2004). Revised guides for organ sampling and trimming in rats and mice – Part 3. Exp. Toxic. Pathol. ,55: 433–449.

Morelli, P., Porazzi, E., Ruspini , M. , Restelli, U., Banfi, G. (2013) . Analysis of errors in histology by root cause analysis: a pilot study. J Prev Med Hyg. , 54 : 90–6. [PMC free article] [PubMed] [Google Scholar]

Mortensen, A.H., Schade, V., Lamonerie, T., Camper, S.A.(2015) . Deletion of OTX2 in neural ectoderm delays anterior pituitary development. Human molecular genetics , 24 : 939-953.

Mosiman, V. L., Patterson, B. K., Canterero, L., and Goolsby, C. L. (1997). Reducing cellular autofluorescence in flow cytometry: an in situ method. Cytometry, 30: 151-156.

Murk, J.L. , Posthuma, G., Koster, A.J. , Geuze, H.J. , Verkleij, A.J. , Kleijmeer, M.J. , Humbel, B.M. (2003) . Influence of aldehyde fixation on the morphology of endosomes and lysosomes : quantitative analysis and electron tomography, J. Microsc. , 212: 81 – 90.

Musumeci, G. (2014) . Past, present and future : overview on Histology and histopathology. J Histol Histopathol., 1: 5. http://dx.doi.org/10.7243/2055-091X-1-5 . [Google Scholar]

Nadworny PL, Wang JF, Tredget EE, Burrell RE (2010) Anti-inflammatory activity of nanocrystalline silver-derived solutions in porcine contact dermatitis. J Inflam. , 7: 13. http://dx.doi.org/10.1186/1476-9255-7-13 .

Nicot, A. S., Toussaint, A., Tosch, V., Kretz, C., Wallgren-Pettersson, C., Iwarsson, E., Kingston, H., Garnier, J. M., Biancalana, V., Oldfors, A. et al. (2007). Mutations in amphiphysin 2 (BIN1) disrupt interaction with dynamin 2 and cause autosomal recessive centronuclear myopathy. Nat. Genet., 39:1134-1139.

Nishi, C. , Nakajima, N., Ikada, Y. (1995). In vitro evaluation of cytotoxicity of diepoxy compounds used for biomaterial modification. J Biomed Mater Res. , 29(7) : 829–834 .

NTP. Addendum to the 12th Report on Carcinogens. USA Department of Health and Human Services, National Toxicology Program, 2011; http://ntp.niehs.nih.gov/ntp/roc/twelfth/Addendum.pdf November 7, 2011 .

Ntziachristos, V. (2010). Going deeper than microscopy: the optical imaging frontier in biology. Nat Methods. , 7: 603 – 614 .http://dx.doi.org/10.1038/nmeth.1483 .

Nuovo, G.J.(1996). Situ hybridization. In: Damjanov I, Linder J, eds. Anderson's Pathology. 10th ed. Maryland Heights , MO : Mosby .

O'Brien, T.P., McCully, M.E. (1981). The Study of Plant Structure : Principles and Selected Methods. 1st ed. Melbourne, Australia: Termarcarphi .

Ortiz-Hidalgo C.(1992) . Pol André Bouin, MD (1870-1962). Bouin's fixative and other contributions to medicine. Arch Pathol Lab Med., 116(8) : 882–884 .

Ortiz-Hidalgo, C. , Pina-Oviedo, S . (2019) . Hematoxylin: Mesoamerica's gift to histopathology. *Palo de Campeche* (logwood tree), pirates' most desired treasure, and irreplaceable tissue stain. Int J Surg Pathol. , 27(1) : 4–14.

OSHA. (Occupational Safety and Health Administration) (2011) Standard Number: 1910.1048 : United States Department of Labor ; http://www.osha.gov/pls/oshaweb/owadisp.show_document?p_id=10075&p_table=STANDARDS November 7, 2011 .

Ozan, G. , Goss, G. (2001) . Gross Dissection and Description . In : National Society for Histotechnology Self-Assessment. No 12.

Paget, E.G., and Thompson, R. (1979) . Standard operating procedures, in Pathology, MTP Press, Lancaster, pp 134–139.

Pfaeffle, R.W., Savage, J.J., Hunter, C.S., Palme, C., Ahlmann, M., Kumar, P., Bellone, J., Schoenau, E., Korsch, E., Bramswig, J.H., Stobbe, H.M., Blum, W.F., Rhodes, S.J. (2007) . Four novel mutations of the LHX3 gene cause combined pituitary hormone deficiencies with or without limited neck rotation. J Clin Endocrinol Metab., 92:1909-1919

Pfaeffle ,R.W., Hunter, C.S., Savage, J.J., Duran-Prado M., Mullen, R.D., Neeb, Z.P., Eiholzer, U., Hesse ,V., Haddad, N.G., Stobbe, H.M., Blum ,W.F., Weigel, J.F., Rhodes, S.J.(2008). Three novel missense mutations within the LHX4 gene are associated with variable pituitary hormone deficiencies. J Clin Endocrinol Metab., 93 : 1062-1071.

Piper, R.C. (1981). Morphological evaluation of the heart in toxicologic studies, in Cardiac toxicology (Balazc, T., ed), Vol. 3, CRC Press, Boca Raton, pp 111–136.

Polishchuk, R.S., Polishchuk, E.V., Marra, P., Alberti, S., Buccione, R., Luini, A., and Mironov, A.A. (2000) . Correlative light-electron microscopy reveals the tubular-saccular ultrastructure of carriers operating between Golgi apparatus and plasma membrane. J. Cell Biol., 148 : 45–58.

Prendergast, G.C., Muller, A.J. , Ramalingam, A. , Chang, M.Y. (2009). BAR the door : cancer suppression by amphiphysin-like genes. Biochim Biophys Acta., 1795 : 25–36.

Prophet, E.B., Mills, B., Sobin, L.H. (eds): (1992). Armed Forces Institute of Pathology Laboratory Methods in Histotechnology . American Registry of Pathology, Washington, DC .

Puchtler, H. , Meloan, S.N., Waldrop, F.S. (1986) . Application of current chemical concepts to metal - haematein and - brazilein stains. Histochemistry, 85: 353–364.

Pulichino, A.M., Vallette-Kasic, S., Couture, C., Gauthier, Y., Brue, T., David, M., Malpuech, G., Deal, C., Van Vliet, G., De Vroede, M., Riepe, F.G., Partsch, C.J., Sippell ,W.G., Berberoglu ,M., Atasay, B., Drouin, J. (2003) . Human and mouse TPIT gene mutations cause early onset pituitary ACTH deficiency. Genes & development, 17:711-716.

Purves, W. K., Sadava, D., Orians, G. H., and Heller, H. C. (2003). Microscopes are needed to visualize cells. In Life: The science of biology (7th ed., pp. 63-64). Sunderland, MA: Sinauer Associates, Inc.

Ramos-Vara, J. A. (2005) Technical Aspects of Immunohistochemistry. Vet. Pathol., **42** : 405-426.

Raven, P. H., Johnson, G. B., Mason, K. A., Losos, J. B., and Singer, S. R. (2014). Cell structure. In Biology (10th ed., AP ed., pp. 59-87). New York, NY: McGraw-Hill.

Reece, J. B., Urry, L. A., Cain, M. L., Wasserman, S. A., Minorsky, P. V., and Jackson, R. B. (2011). A tour of the cell. In Campbell Biology (10th ed., pp. 92-123). San Francisco, CA: Pearson.

Rodrigues, E. B., Costa, E. F., Penha, Fm. M., Melo, G. B. , Bottós, J., Dib, E., Farah, M. E. (2009) . The use of vital dyes in ocular surgery.

Survey of Ophthalmology., 54(5) : 576–617. http://dx.doi.org/10.1016/j.survophthal.2009.04.011 . [PubMed] [Google Scholar]

Rolls, G.O., Farmer, N. J., Hall, J.B. (2008) . Artifacts in Histological and Cytological Preparations. Melbourne: Leica Microsystems, 106.

Rolls ,G. (2008). 101 Steps to Better Histology. Melbourne: Leica Microsystems,

Rolls, G.O., Farmer, N.J., Hall, J.B. (1994). Artefacts in histological and cytological preparations. In Woods A and Ellis R eds. Laboratory histopathology. New York: Churchill Livingstone, 5.3-1 - 5.3-29.

Herms J. R., Johanna F.M. van Uum. , Ingrid, B. , Jasper E., Radu L., and Chris W. Pool. (1999). Double Immunolabeling of Neuropeptides in the Human Hypothalamus as Analyzed by Confocal Laser Scanning Fluorescence Microscopy. Journal of Histochemistry and Cytochemistry , 47: 229-236.

Rotimi, O., Cairns,. A, Gray ,S., Moayyedi, P., Dixon, M. F. (2000) . Histological identification of Helicobacter pylori : comparison of staining methods. [Retrieved August 18, 2014 from] ; J Clin Pathol., 53 : 756 – 759. http://dx.doi.org/10.1136/jcp.53.10.756 .

Rudijanto, A. (2007) . The role of vascular smooth muscle cells on the pathogenesis of atherosclerosis. Acta Med Indones , 39 : 86–93.

Ruehl-Fehlert, C., Kittel, B., Morawietz, G., Deslex, P., Keenan, C., Mahrt, C.R., Nolte, T., Robinson, M., Stuart, B.P., and Deschl, U. (2003). Revised guides for organ sampling and trimming in rats and mice – Part 1. Exp. Toxic. Pathol. , 55: 91–106.

Russell , D. G. , Gordon, S. (2009) . Phagocyte-pathogen interactions: macrophages and the host response to infection. Washington, D.C: ASM Press.

Sabatini, D.D. , Bensch, K. , Barrnett, R.J. (1963) . Cytochemistry and electron microscopy. The preservation of cellular ultrastructure and enzymatic activity by aldehyde fixation. J Cell Biol. , 17 : 19–58 .

Santoianni, R.A., Hammami, A . (1990) . Nuclear Bubbling an Overlooked Artifact. The Journal of Histotechnology, 13 : 135-136.

Sartori, A. , Gatz, R., Beck, F., Rigort, A. , Baumeister W, Plitzko, J.M. (2007) . Correlative microscopy: bridging the gap between fluorescence light microscopy and cryo-electron tomography. J Struct Biol., 160: 135–145.

Sawaguchi, A. , Yao, X. , Forte, J.G., McDonald, K.L. (2003). Direct attachment of cell suspensions to high-pressure freezing specimen planchettes. J Microsc., 212 : 13–20.

Schaletzky, J. , Dove, S.K. , Short, B., Lorenzo, O. , Clague, M.J. , and Barr, F.A. (2003) . Phosphatidylinositol-5-phosphate activation and conserved substrate specificity of the myotubularin phosphatidylinositol 3-phosphatases. Curr Biol. , 13 : 504–509.

Schwarz, H., Humbel, B.M. (2007). Correlative light and electron microscopy using immunolabeled resin sections. Methods Mol Biol., 369 : 229–256 .

Sheehan, D.C. , and Hrapchak, B.B. (1980) . Theory and Practice of Histotechnology. 2nd Ed., Battelle Press, Ohio .

Sheehan, D.C., Hrapchak, B.B. (1987) . Theory and Practice of Histotechnology. 2nd ed. Battelle Press . , Columbus , OH .

Shi, Z. R., Itzkowitz, S. H., Kim, Y. S. (1988) . A comparison of three immunoperoxidase techniques for antigen detection in colorectal carcinoma tissues. J. Histochem. Cytochem. , 36 : 317-322 .

Shinoda, K., Lei, H., Yoshii, H., Nomura, M., Nagano, M., Shiba, H., Sasaki, H., Osawa, Y., Ninomiya ,Y., Niwa, O. (1995) . Developmental defects of the ventromedial hypothalamic nucleus and pituitary gonadotroph in the Ftz-F1 disrupted mice. Developmental dynamics , 204 : 22-29.

Shoja, M.M., Tubbs, R.S., Loukas, M., Shokouhi, G., Ardalan, M.R. (2008). Marie-François Xavier Bichat (1771-1802) and his contributions to the foundations of pathological anatomy and modern medicine. Ann Anat., 190 (5) : 413-420. doi:10.1016/j.aanat..07.004

Snabboon ,T. , Plengpanich, W. , Buranasupkajorn, P. , Khwanjaipanich, R. , Vasinanukorn, P. , Suwanwalaikorn, S. , Khovidhunkit, W. , Shotelersuk, V. (2008) . A novel germline mutation, IVS4+1G>A, of the POU1F1 gene underlying combined pituitary hormone deficiency. Horm Res., 69 : 60-64.

Spillan ,B.S. (1976) . Proper Tissue Embedding Practices. Histologic Magazine. , VI(2) : 79.

Spurr, A.R. (1969) . A low-viscosity epoxy resin embedding medium for electron microscopy, Journal of Ultrastructure Research, 26(1-2) : 31-43 .

Stickrod, G. and Stansifer, M. (1981)"Perfusion of Small Animals Using a Mini-Peristaltic Pump," Physiol. Behav. , 27(6) : 1127-1128,.

Studer, D., Humbel, B.M., Chiquet, M. (2008). Electron microscopy of high pressure frozen samples: bridging the gap between cellular ultrastructure and atomic resolution. Histochem Cell Biol ., 130 : 877–889.

Suh, H. , Gage, P.J. , Drouin, J. , Camper, S.A. (2002) . Pitx2 is required at multiple stages of pituitary organogenesis: pituitary primordium formation and cell specification. Development., 129 : 329-337.

Sung, H.W., Liang, I.L., Chen, C.N., Huang, R.N., Liang, H.F. (2001) . Stability of a biological tissue fixed with a naturally occurring crosslinking agent (genipin) . J Biomed Mater Res., 55(4) : 538–546

Sung, H.W., Huang, R.N., Huang, L.L., Tsai, C.C. (1999). In vitro evaluation of cytotoxicity of a naturally occurring cross-linking reagent for biological tissue fixation. J Biomater Sci Polym Ed., 10(1) : 63–78

Sung, H.W., Chang, Y., Liang, I.L., Chang, W.H., Chen ,Y.C. (2000) . Fixation of biological tissues with a naturally occurring crosslinking agent: fixation rate and effects of pH, temperature, and initial fixative concentration. J Biomed Mater Res., 52(1) : 77–87 .

Suvarna, S. K., Layton, C., Bancroft, J.D. (2013) . Bancroft's Theory and practice of Histological techniques, Expert consult . 7th Edition. Churchill Livingstone, Elsevier.

Taber's Cyclopedic Medical Dictionary. (2005) . 21st ed. Philadelphia, PA: FA Davis Co.

Tajima, T., Ishizu, K., Nakamura, A. (2013). Molecular and Clinical Findings in Patients with LHX4 and OTX2 Mutations. Clinical pediatric endocrinology : case reports and clinical investigations : official journal of the Japanese Society for Pediatric Endocrinology, 22:15-23.

Thomson-Russell, K.C. and Edington, J.W. (1977). Electron Microscope preparation techniques in material science. Macmillan Ed.

Thompson, S.W. and Luna, L.G. (1978). An Atlas of Artifacts of Artifacts Encountered in the Preparation of Microscopic Tissue Sections. Charles C. Thomas Publisher, Springfield, IL .

Thornthwaite, J.T. , Thomas ,R.A. , Leif, S.B. , Yopp, T.A. et al. (1978) . The use of electronic cell volume analysis with the AMAC II to determine the optimum glutaraldehyde fixative concentration for nucleated mammalian cells. Scan Electron Microscopy, 2 : 1123.

Titford, M.E., Horenstein ,M. G. (2005) . Histomorphologic assessment of formalin substitute fixatives for diagnostic surgical pathology. Arch Pathol Lab Med., 129(4) : 502–506.

Titford, M. A. (2006) . Short History of Histopathology Technique. J Histotechnol., 29(2) : 99-110. doi:10.1179/his.2006.29.2.99.

Titford, M. (2009) . Progress in the development of microscopical techniques for diagnostic pathology. J.Histotechnol. , 32 : 9 – 19. http://dx.doi.org/10.1179/his.2009.32.1.9 .

Titford, M. , Bowman, B. (2012) . What May the Future Hold for Histotechnologists? LabMedicine. , 43 : 5–10.

TEM specimen preparation techniques D. V. Sridhara Rao, K. Muraleedharan, and C. J. Humphreys Microscopy: Science, Technology,

Applications and Education, Volume-2, A. Méndez-Vilas and J. Díaz (Eds.), 2010.

Tokuyasu, K.T .(1973). A technique for ultracryotomy of cell suspensions and tissues. J Cell Biol., 57: 551–565.

Treier, M. , Gleiberman, A.S., O'Connell, S.M., Szeto, D.P., McMahon ,J.A., McMahon, A.P., Rosenfeld, M.G.(1998) . Multistep signaling requirements for pituitary organogenesis in vivo. Genes & development., 12:1691-1704.

Treier, M., O'Connell, S., Gleiberman, A., Price, J., Szeto, D.P., Burgess, R., Chuang, P.T., McMahon, A.P., Rosenfeld, M.G.(2001). Hedgehog signaling is required for pituitary gland development. Development . , 128 : 377-386.

Turton ,J.P., Mehta, A., Raza, J., Woods, K.S., Tiulpakov, A., Cassar, J., Chong, K., Thomas, P.Q., Eunice , M., Ammini, A.C., Bouloux, P.M., Starzyk, J. , Hindmarsh, P.C., Dattani, M.T.(2005). Mutations within the transcription factor PROP1 are rare in a cohort of patients with sporadic combined pituitary hormone deficiency (CPHD). Clin Endocrinol (Oxf) . , 63:10-18.

Vallette-Kasic ,S. , Brue, T., Pulichino, A.M., Gueydan, M., Barlier, A., David, M., Nicolino, M., Malpuech, G., Dechelotte, P., Deal, C., Van Vliet, G., De Vroede, M., Riepe, F.G., Partsch, C.J., Sippell, W.G., Berberoglu, M., Atasay, B., de Zegher, F., Beckers, D., Kyllo, J., Donohoue, P., Fassnacht, M., Hahner, S., Allolio ,B., Noordam, C., Dunkel, L., Hero , M. , Pigeon, B. , Weill, J. , Yigit, S., Brauner, R., Heinrich, J.J., Cummings, E., Riddell, C. , Enjalbert ,A., Drouin, J. (2005) . Congenital isolated deficiency: an underestimated cause of neonatal death, explained by TPIT gene mutations. J Clin Endocrinol Metab. , 90 : 1323-1331.

Vander Voort, G. F. (2004) ed., "Chemical and Electrolytic Polishing," ASM Handbook, Vol. 9: Metallography and Microstructures, ASM International , p 281-293,

ISBN 978-0-87170-706-2.

van der Laak, J.A.W.M. , Pahlplatz , M.M.M. , Hanselaar, A.G.J.M., de Wilde, P.C.M. (2000) . Hue-saturation density (HSD) model for stain transmitted light microscopy. Cytometry. , 39:275–284.

van Rijnsoever, C., Oorschot, V., Klumperman, J. (2008). Correlative light-electron microscopy (CLEM) combining live-cell imaging and immunolabeling of ultrathin cryosections. Nat Methods, 5: 973–980.

Verkade, P. (2008). Moving EM: the Rapid Transfer System as a new tool for correlative light and electron microscopy and high throughput for high-pressure freezing. J Microsc ., 230 : 317–328.

Vicidomini ,G., Gagliani , M.C., Canfora , M. , Cortese, K., Frosi, F., Santangelo , C. , Di Fiore, P. , et al. (2008) . High data output and automated 3D correlative light-electron microscopy method. Traffic, 9: 1828–1838.

Victor, B. (2013) . Histological techniques for life science researchers. . [Retrieved August 18, 2014
from].http://www.slideshare.net/biotechvictor1950/histological-techniques.

Vieira ,T.C., Boldarine, V.T., Abucham, J. (2007). Molecular analysis of PROP1, PIT1, HESX1, LHX3, and LHX4 shows high frequency of PROP1 mutations in patients with familial forms of combined pituitary hormone deficiency. Arquivos brasileiros de endocrinologia e metabologia ., 51:1097-1103.

Walck, S.D. , McCaffrey, J.P. (1997) . in: R.M. Anderson, S.D.Walek (Eds.),Specimen Preparation for Transmission Electron Microscopy of Materials IV, Vol. 480, Materials Research Society, Pittsburgh, PA, , p. 149.

Walker, W. F. (1980). Vertebrate dissection. Sixth Ed, W.B. Saunders Comp. Philadelphia.

Walker, J.F. (1964) . Formaldehyde. 3rd ed. American Chemical Society Monograph Series. Reinhold Publishing , New York, NY.

Weaver, J. (2010) . Paraffin Embedding and Process Improvement. Presented by Teleconference Network of Texas, UT Health Science Center

Weiss, A. T. , Delcour, N. M. , Meyer, A., Klopfleisch, R. (2010) . Efficient Cost-Effective Extraction of Genomic DNA from Formalin-Fixed and Paraffin-Embedded Tissues. Veterinary Pathology, 22(4) : 834–838.

West, J.B. (2013) . Marcello Malpighi and the discovery of the pulmonary capillaries and alveoli. Am J Physiol Lung Cell Mol Physiol. , 304(6) : L383-90. doi:10.1152/ajplung.00016.2013.

Westra, W.H., Hruban , R.H., Phelps, T.H., Isacson, C. (2009) . Surgical Pathology Dissection: An Illustrated Guide. 2nd ed. , Springer-Verlag , New York, NY .

Wicks , L. F., Suntzeff, V. (1943) . Glyoxal, a non-irritating aldehyde suggested as substitute for formalin in histological fixations. Science , 982539 : 204.

Williams , D. B and Carter, C. B. (1996) . Transmission Electron Microscopy, Plenum Press, New York .

Windsor, L. (1994). Tissue processing , in Laboratory histopathology, a complete reference (Woods, A.E., and Ellis, R.C., eds), Churchill Livingstone, New York, Vol. 1, pp 4.2-1/4.2-42.

World Health Organization. Concise International Chemical Assessment Document 57 GLYOXAL. 2004;

http://whqlibdoc.who.int/publications/2004/924153057X.pdf; November 22'

Yan , L.P., Wang ,Y.J. , Ren, L., Wu,G., Caridade,S.G., Fan,J.B., Wang, L.Y., Ji,P.H., Oliveira, J. M., Oliveira,J.O.T., Mano, J.O.F., Rui L. Reis, R.L..(2010). Genipin-cross-linked collagen/chitosan biomimetic scaffolds for articular cartilage tissue engineering applications. J Biomed Mater Res A., 95(2) : 465–475 .

Young ,D.G. (2001). An easy and effective quality monitoring system for H&E staining. J Histotechnol. , 24(2):125–127.

Young, B., O'Dowd, G., Stewart, W., Paul R .W. (2010). Wheater's Basic Pathology: A Text, Atlas and Review of Histopathology. 5th Ed. , Churchill Livingstone, Edinburgh .

Zhu, X., Gleiberman, A.S., Rosenfeld, M.G.(2007) . Molecular physiology of pituitary development: signaling and transcriptional networks. Physiological reviews , 87:933-963.

Zwienenberg , M., Gong, Q., Lee, L. L., Berman, R. F., Lyeth, B. G. J. (1999). Neurotrauma. Monitoring in the Rat: Comparison of Monitoring in the Ventricle, Brain Parenchyma, and Cisterna Magna. , 16:1095-1102 .

MANUAL OF HISTOLOGICAL TECHNIQUES AND AN ATLAS OF HISTOLOGY AND ULTRASTRUCTURAL DETAILS OF SOME ENDOCRINE GLANDS

GLOSSARY

Acid : A substance that increases the hydrogen ion concentration of a solution.

Acid dye : A dye in which the colored component is an anion, e.g. Congo red and eosin Y. Such dyes are not acids, the term derives from 19th century textile dyeing, when they are used to color silk and wool from acid dyebaths.

Acidophilic : Literally, acid [dye] loving. Usually proteins, which take up acid dyes. Examples of acidophilic tissue components are collagen fibres, nuclear histones and erythrocytes.

Acrosome : (ak_-ruh-so–m) A vesicle in the tip of a sperm containing hydrolytic enzymes and other proteins that help the sperm reach the egg.

Adipose tissue : A connective tissue that insulates the body and serves as a fuel reserve; contains fat-storing cells called adipose cells.

Adrenal gland : (uh-dre‾_-nul) One of two endocrine glands located adjacent to the kidneys in mammals. Endocrine cells in the outer portion (cortex) respond to adrenocorticotropic hormone (ACTH) by secreting steroid hormones that help maintain homeostasis during long-term stress. Neurosecretory cells in the central portion (medulla) secrete epinephrine and norepinephrine in response to nerve signals triggered by short-term stress.

Adrenocorticotropic hormone (ACTH) : A tropic hormone that is produced and secreted by the anterior pituitary and that stimulates the production and secretion of steroid hormones by the adrenal cortex.

Aldosterone : (al-dos_-tuh-ro–n) A steroid hormone that acts on tubules of the kidney to regulate the transport of sodium ions (Na_) and potassium ions (K_).

amino acid : (uh-mē n̄-o–) An organic molecule possessing both a carboxyl and an amino group. Amino acids serve as the monomers of polypeptides.

amino group : A chemical group consisting of a nitrogen atom bonded to two hydrogen atoms; can act as a base in solution, accepting a hydrogen ion and acquiring a charge of 1_.

anatomy : The structure of an organism.

androgen : (an_-dro–-jen) Any steroid hormone, such as testosterone, that stimulates the development and maintenance of the male reproductive system and secondary sex characteristics.

angiotensin II : A peptide hormone that stimulates constriction of precapillary arterioles and increases reabsorption of NaCl and water by the proximal tubules of the kidney, increasing blood pressure and volume.

anion : (an_-ī̄-on) A negatively charged ion.

Anion, Anionic : A negatively charged atom or molecule, for instance an ionic species such as an acid dye or a chloride ion. Anions are attracted to the positive electrode (anode) in electrophoresis.

Anterior : Pertaining to the front, or head, of a bilaterally symmetrical animal.

anterior pituitary : A portion of the pituitary that develops from non neural tissue; consists of endocrine cells that synthesize and secrete several tropic and nontropic hormones.

antidiuretic hormone (ADH) : (an_-tī̄-dī̄-yū̄- ret_-ik) A peptide hormone, also known as vasopressin, that promotes water retention by the kidneys. Produced in the hypothalamus and released from the posterior pituitary, ADH also functions in the brain.

apocrine : a form of secretion in which a portion of the cytoplasm leaves the cell together with the product of secretion.

apoptosis : programmed cell death (carefully orchestrated by genes and gene products that turn the pathway to cell death on or off) ; fragmentation of the cell into membrane-bound particles that are eliminated by phagocytosis ; from the Greek for "falling off".

arteriole : (ar-ter̄-ē-o–l) A vessel that conveys blood between an artery and a capillary bed.

artery : A vessel that carries blood away from the heart to organs throughout the body.

astrocyte : A glial cell with diverse functions, including providing structural support for neurons, regulating the interstitial environment, facilitating synaptic transmission, and assisting in regulating the blood supply to the brain.

ATP (adenosine triphosphate) : (a-den̄-o–-sēn trī-fos̄-fa–t) An adenine-containing nucleoside triphosphate that releases free energy when its phosphate bonds are hydrolyzed. This energy is used to drive endergonic reactions in cells.

ATP synthase : A complex of several membrane proteins that functions in chemiosmosis with adjacent electron transport chains, using the energy of a hydrogen ion (proton) concentration gradient to make ATP. ATP synthases are found in the inner mitochondrial membranes of eukaryotic cells and in the plasma membranes of prokaryotes.

atrial natriuretic peptide (ANP) : (a–̄-trē-ul nā-trē-yū-retˉ-ik) A peptide hormone secreted by cells of the atria of the heart in response to high blood pressure. ANP's effects on the kidney alter ion and water movement and reduce blood pressure.

Autocrine : Referring to a secreted molecule that acts on the cell that secreted it.

B cells : The lymphocytes that complete their development in the bone marrow and become effector cells for the humoral immune response.

Base : A substance that reduces the hydrogen ion concentration of a solution.

Basic dye : A dye with a cationic colored component, e.g. alcian blue, hemalum, or neutral red. Such basic dyes are not bases; the term derives from textile dyeing usage, in which they were originally used to color silk and wool fibres from alkaline ("basic") dyebaths.

Basophil.: A type of leukocyte with large basophilic cytoplasmic granules.

Basophilia, basophilic : (1) Literally, basic dye lover. Basophilic tissue components, with affinity for basic dyes, include cartilage matrix, nuclear chromatin, and mast cell granules. **(2)** In hematology, basophilia means an abnormally large number of basophil leukocytes in the blood, traditionally determined by counting cell types in a Romanowsky stained blood film.

bile : A mixture of substances that is produced in the liver and stored in the gallbladder; enables formation of fat droplets in water as an aid in the digestion and absorption of fats.

Biotechnology : The manipulation of organisms or their components to produce useful products.

Blood : A connective tissue with a fluid matrix called plasma in which red blood cells, white blood cells, and cell fragments called platelets are suspended.

body cavity : A fluid- or air-filled space between the digestive tract and the body wall.

Bouin's fluid : A rationally contrived fixative mixture of three ingredients that can stabilize an immersed animal tissue in different ways. Formaldehyde penetrates quickly and modifies proteins. Acetic acid enters cells and their nuclei, precipitating chromatin . Picric acid coagulates proteins and also opposes the tissue swelling caused by acetic acid.

Bowman's capsule : (bo–_-munz) A cup-shaped receptacle in the vertebrate kidney that is the initial, expanded segment of the nephron where filtrate enters from the blood.

brain : Organ of the central nervous system where information is processed and integrated.

brainstem : A collection of structures in the vertebrate brain, including the midbrain, the pons, and the medulla oblongata; functions in homeostasis, coordination of movement, and conduction of information to higher brain centers.

Buffer : A solution that maintains a constant pH after addition of small amounts of acid or base. It is typically made of a salt and a weak acid, which are in equilibrium in the solution. If additional hydrogen ions (more acid) are added, they combine with the base of the salt. If more alkali (OH$^-$) is added, it neutralizes the weak acid. In either case, the pH does not change. Specific buffer solutions maintain pH over limited ranges, typically about 2 pH units.

Calcitonin : (kal_-si-to–_-nin) A hormone secreted by the thyroid gland that lowers blood calcium levels by promoting calcium deposition in bone and calcium excretion from the kidneys; nonessential in adult humans.

carbohydrate : (kar_-bo–hī̄_-dra–t) A sugar (monosaccharide) or one of its dimers (disaccharides) or polymers (polysaccharides).

Catecholamine : (kat_-uh-ko–l_-uh-mē̄n) Any of a class of neurotransmitters and hormones, including the hormones epinephrine and norepinephrine, that are synthesized from the amino acid tyrosine.

Cell : the fundamental unit of life.

Cell Membrane : a thin semi-permeable membrane that surrounds the cytoplasm of a cell.

Chromatin : the mass of genetic material composed of DNA and proteins that condense to form chromosomes during eukaryotic cell division.

Chromosome : a long, stringy aggregate of genes that carries heredity information (DNA) and is formed from condensed chromatin.

Celsius scale : (sel_-sē̄-us) A temperature scale (°C) equal to 5/9(°F – 32) that measures the freezing point of water at 0°C and the boiling point of water at 100°C.

central canal : The narrow cavity in the center of the spinal cord that is continuous with the fluid-filled ventricles of the brain.

central nervous system (CNS) : The portion of the nervous system where signal integration occurs; in vertebrate animals, the brain and spinal cord.

cerebellum : (sa–r_-ruh-bel_-um) Part of the vertebrate hindbrain located dorsally ; functions in unconscious coordination of movement and balance.

Cervix : (ser_-viks) The neck of the uterus, which opens into the vagina.

Chelating agent : Some are mordant dyes which react with metal ions giving rise to stains. Examples include carminic acid, celestine blue, gallocyanine, hematein and nuclear fast red. Some are used to generate colored products from tissue constituents, e.g.: demonstration of calcium ions by chelation with alizarin red S; or of nickel ions by chelation with dimethylglyoxime. Another chelating agent, EDTA, is used for decalcification of tissues.

Chelation : Formation of a metal coordination complex by the reaction of a metal ion with a chelating agent. This involves a compound carrying two or more metal binding groups (such as CO_2^-, OH or C=O), which are able to form a complete covalently bonded ring that includes the metal ion. Such chelate rings often are chemically stable structures.

chemoreceptor : A sensory receptor that responds to a chemical stimulus, such as a solute or an odorant.

cholesterol : (ko– -les̄-tuh-rol) A steroid that forms n essential component of animal cell membranes and acts as a precursor molecule for the synthesis of other biologically important steroids, such as many hormones.

chromosome : (kro–̄-muh-so–m) A cellular structure carrying genetic material, found in the nucleus of eukaryotic cells. Each chromosome consists of one very long DNA molecule and associated proteins. (A bacterial chromosome usually consists of a single circular DNA molecule and associated proteins. It is found in the nucleoid region, which is not membrane bounded.) *See also* chromatin.

Chromatin : the mass of genetic material composed of DNA and proteins that condense to form chromosomes during eukaryotic cell division.

circadian rhythm : (ser-ka–̄-dē -un) A physiological cycle of about 24 hours that persists even in the absence of external cues.

Clearing agent. : A solvent used to remove the dehydrant and unbound lipids from a tissue specimen during tissue processing, and to prepare the specimen for immersion into paraffin wax; typically an aromatic hydrocarbon (xylene or toluene), an aliphatic hydrocarbon (various proprietary mixtures), or d-limonene. Clearing agents are also used to remove wax from sections prior to staining, and to remove the dehyrant from sections prior to coverslipping with a non-aqueous mounting medium.

clitoris : (klit̄-uh-ris) An organ at the upper intersection of the labia minora that engorges with blood and becomes erect during sexual arousal.

Coelom : (sē̄ -lo–m) A body cavity lined by tissue derived only from mesoderm.

collagen : A glycoprotein in the extracellular matrix of animal cells that forms strong fibers, found extensively in connective tissue and bone; the most abundant protein in the animal kingdom.

collecting duct : The location in the kidney where processed filtrate, called urine, is collected from the renal tubules.

columnar (cells) : - refers to a shape of cells which often line ducts or glands within the body.

Compound : A substance consisting of two or more different elements combined in a fixed ratio.

connective tissue : Animal tissue that functions mainly to bind and support other tissues, having a sparse population of cells scattered through an extracellular matrix.

corpus luteum : (kor_-pus lu¯_-te¯-um) A secreting tissue in the ovary that forms from the collapsed follicle after ovulation and produces progesterone.

cortex : (1) The outer region of cytoplasm in a eukaryotic cell, lying just under the plasma membrane,that has a more gel-like consistency than the inner regions due to the presence of multiple microfilaments. (2) In plants, ground tissue that is between the vascular tissue and dermal tissue in a root or eudicot stem.

cortical nephron : In mammals and birds, a nephron with a loop of Henle located almost entirely in the renal cortex.

corticosteroid : Any steroid hormone produced and secreted by the adrenal cortex.

crista (plural, **cristae**) : (kris_-tuh, kris_-te¯) An infolding of the inner membrane of a mitochondrion.The inner membrane houses electron transport chains and molecules of the enzyme catalyzing the synthesis of ATP (ATP synthase).

cytoplasm : (si¯_-to--plaz_-um) The contents of the cell bounded by the plasma membrane; in eukaryotes, the portion exclusive of the nucleus.

cytotoxic T cell : A type of lymphocyte that, when activated, kills infected cells as well as certain cancer cells and transplanted cells.

Delafield's hematoxylin : A *regressive* version of *hemalum* containing *hematoxylin* and aluminium ammonium sulfate, as well as water and ethanol as solvents and glycerol as a stabilizer to prevent over-oxidation. The solution is oxidized slowly by air and sunlight over a period of months.

dendrite (den_-drī t) One of usually numerous, short, highly branched extensions of a neuron that receive signals from other neurons.

diabetes mellitus (dī_-uh-bē_-tis mel_-uh-tus) An endocrine disorder marked by an inability to maintain glucose homeostasis. The type 1 form results from autoimmune destruction of insulin-secreting cells; treatment usually requires daily insulin injections. The type 2 form most commonly results from reduced responsiveness of target cells to insulin; obesity and lack of exercise are risk factors.

Differential stain. A solution of variously colored dyes with selective affinities for different tissue components (e.g., Romanowsky stains, trichrome mixtures.

Differentiation. In histotechnical usage: controlled de-staining of a stained section.

distal tubule In the vertebrate kidney, the portion of a nephron that helps refine filtrate and empties it into a collecting duct.

disulfide bridge A strong covalent bond formed when the sulfur of one cysteine monomer bonds to the sulfur of another cysteine monomer.

dopamine A neurotransmitter that is a catecholamine, like epinephrine and norepinephrine.

electron A subatomic particle with a single negative electrical charge and a mass about 1/2,000 that of a neutron or proton. One or more electrons move around the nucleus of an atom. Electrons and their orbits around the nucleus of an atom account for most of the physical properties of the element. Used extensively in Electron Microscopy.

Electron Gun A cathode/anode device intended to produce a stream of electrons. A more detailed explination and diagram is available.

electron microscope (EM) A microscope that uses magnets to focus an electron beam on or through a specimen, resulting in a practical resolution of a hundredfold greater than that of a light microscope using standard techniques. A transmission electron microscope (TEM) is used to study the internal structure of thin sections of cells. A scanning electron microscope (SEM) is used to study the fine details of cell surfaces.

Electron microscopy (EM). The study of the ultrastructure of specimens, biological or otherwise, using an electron microscope.

Embedding. Cells and tissues are immersed in a liquid, such as molten paraffin wax or the monomer of a plastic embedding medium. After the liquid is solidified, by freezing or polymerization respectively, the embedded specimen is interpenetrated and supported by a solid matrix, the **embedding medium**.

endocrine gland (en_-do--krin) A ductless gland that secretes hormones directly into the interstitial fluid, from which they diffuse into the bloodstream.

endocrine system The internal system of communication involving hormones, the ductless glands that secrete hormones, and the molecular receptors on or in target cells that respond to hormones; functions in concert with the nervous system to effect internal regulation and maintain homeostasis.

endocytosis (en_-do- -sī -to-_-sis) Cellular uptake of biological molecules and particulate matter via formation of vesicles from the plasma membrane.

endoderm (en_-do--durm) The innermost of the three primary germ layers in animal embryos; lines the archenteron and gives rise to the liver, pancreas, lungs, and the lining of the digestive tract in species that have these structures.

endometrium (en_-do--mē_-trē-um) The inner lining of the uterus, which is richly supplied with blood vessels.

endoplasmic reticulum (ER) (en_-do--plaz_-mik ruh-tik_-yū-lum) An extensive membranous network in eukaryotic cells, continuous with the outer nuclear membrane and composed of ribosome-studded (rough) and ribosome-free (smooth) regions. It helps in control of protein synthesis and cellular organization.

eosin - any of a class of rose-colored stains or dyes; bromine derivatives of fluorescein; used in histology as a stain.

Eosin B. A moderately large, hydrophilic dibromodinitrofluorescein (i.e. xanthene) acid dye. Sometimes used as the counterstain in Romanowsky stains, and originally specified as such for the Leishman and Wright variants. The dye is soluble in water and ethanol. Synonyms: 45400, Acid red 91. Commercial lots are available certified by the Biological Stain Commission.

Eosin Y. A moderately large tetrabromofluorescein (i.e. xanthene) acid dye. This dye is widely used in histology, notably in the hematoxylin and eosin, Papanicolaou and Romanowsky stains. Also used to stain various acidophilic structures such as eosinophil granules and Negri bodies; and as a cytoplasmic counterstain in various procedures, such as silver stains. Eosin Y is soluble in water, but poorly soluble in alcohol except under acidic conditions. Synonyms: CI 45380, Acid Red 87, eosin. Commercial lots are available in a fairly pure form certified by the Biological Stain Commission.

epididymis (ep_-uh-did_-uh-mus) A coiled tubule located adjacent to the mammalian testis where sperm are stored.

epinephrine (ep_-i-nef_-rin) A catecholamine that, when secreted as a hormone by the adrenal medulla, mediates "fight-or-flight" responses to short-term stresses; also released by some neurons as a neurotransmitter; also known as adrenaline.

epithelial tissue (ep_-uh-the͞_-le͞_-ul) Sheets of tightly packed cells that line organs and body cavities as well as external surfaces.

epithelium An epithelial tissue.

estradiol (es_-truh-dı͞_-ol) A steroid hormone that stimulates the development and maintenance of the female reproductive system and secondary sex characteristics; the major estrogen in mammals.

estrogen (es_-tro--jen) Any steroid hormone, such as estradiol, that stimulates the development and maintenance of the female reproductive system and secondary sex characteristics.

estrous cycle (es_-trus) A reproductive cycle characteristic of female mammals except humans and certain other primates, in which the nonpregnant endometrium is reabsorbed rather than shed, and sexual response occurs only during mid-cycle at estrus.

euchromatin (yu͞_-kro-_-muh-tin) The less condensed form of eukaryotic chromatin that is available for transcription.

eukaryotic cell (yu͞_-ker-e͞_-ot_-ik) A type of cell with a membrane-enclosed nucleus and membrane-enclosed organelles. Organisms with eukaryotic cells (protists, plants, fungi, and animals) are called eukaryotes.

Fixation. This involves transformation of constituents of cells and tissues into insoluble forms no longer subject to dissolution, destruction by endogenous enzymes (autolysis) or destruction by exogenous enzymes (microbial decomposition). This preserves the native morphology and chemical reactivity of the biological specimen during processing, staining, and microscopic observation. Mechanistically, fixation is complex, and may involve crosslinking of biopolymers and unsaturated lipids, denaturation of proteins resulting in hydrophobic inversion, and trapping of nucleic acids, polysaccharides and some small molecules within a mesh of fixed proteins.

Fixatives. Reagents used to achieve cell and tissue fixation. Common fixatives are reactive aldehydes or other small molecule organic compounds, e.g. formaldehyde, glyoxal, glutaraldehyde or picric acid; reactive metal ions or derivatives, e.g. $Cr_2O_{72}^-$, Hg^{2+}, OsO_4, Zn^{2+}; or organic solvents such as acetic acid, acetone, ethanol or methanol. Most fixatives are protein denaturants and some also form crosslinks. Solvents less polar than water cause hydrophobic inversions. Many useful fixatives are mixtures of compounds with different actions, such as combinations of formaldehyde (a crosslinker) with protein precipitants such as ethanol, picric acid or a zinc salt.

follicle (fol_-uh-kul) A microscopic structure in he ovary that contains the developing oocyte and secretes estrogens.

follicle-stimulating hormone (FSH) A tropic hormone that is produced and secreted by the anterior pituitary and that stimulates the production of eggs by the ovaries and sperm by the testes.

Formaldehyde. A gas (CH_2=O), typically sold as formalin, a 40% w/v (37% w/w) solution in water, with methanol added to inhibit formation of paraformaldehyde. Formaldehyde is the active ingredient in many fixatives.

Formaldehyde fixation. Given sufficient time, formaldehyde fixes tissue first by addition to form hydroxymethyl adducts, and subsequently by crosslinking via methylene bridges. The latter process may continue for many months. Tissue groups attacked by formaldehyde include amides, amines (primary and secondary), hydroxyls, reactive hydrogen atoms on aromatic amino acids, and sulfhydryls.

Formalin. A concentrated solution (37% w/w or 40% w/v) of formaldehyde in water, usually with 10-15% methanol to inhibit polymerization. Synonym: formol. So-called "10% formalin" is a 10% v/v dilution containing 4% w/v formaldehyde. This is the most common fixative for specimens taken from animals and people. The dilution is usually into either saline or a sodium phosphate buffer at neutral pH that is approximately isotonic with extracellular fluids.

gall bladder An organ that stores bile and releases it as needed into the small intestine.

glomerulus (glo–-ma–r_-yu‾ -lus) A ball of capillaries surrounded by Bowman's capsule in the nephron and serving as the site of filtration in the vertebrate kidney.

glucagon (glu‾ _-kuh-gon) A hormone secreted by pancreatic alpha cells that raises blood glucose levels. It promotes glycogen breakdown and release of glucose by the liver.

glucocorticoid A steroid hormone that is secreted by the adrenal cortex and that influences glucose metabolism and immune function.

Glutaraldehyde. $O=CH(CH_2)_3CH=O$. A *fixative* for electron microscopy that *crosslinks* proteins and polyhydroxy (carbohydrate) materials.

glycogen (glı‾ _-ko–-jen) An extensively branched glucose storage polysaccharide found in the liver and muscle of animals; the animal equivalent of starch.

glycolipid A lipid with one or more covalently attached carbohydrates.

Golgi. Camillo Golgi (1843–1926) was an Italian pathologist and histologist. He experimented with silver staining and, in 1873, noticed blackening of occasional whole neurons in pieces of nervous tissue that had been stored in potassium dichromate solution (a commonly used fixative at the time) and then immersed in a solution of silver nitrate. He used this method to describe sensory organs in tendons and various types of neurons in the brain, which are associated with his name. In 1898, using a similar method, he described the "internal reticular apparatus", now known as the Golgi complex and recognized as an organelle present in all eukaryotic cells. Golgi shared the Nobel Prize in Physiology or Medicine with Ramon y Cajal, in 1906.

Golgi staining. A group of methods in which pieces of central nervous tissue are sequentially immersed in solutions of potassium dichromate and silver nitrate. Black deposits of silver chromate are precipitated within the cytoplasm of a small proportion of cells, displaying especially the dendrites of neurons and cytoplasmic processes of glial cells.

Golgi-Cox stain. A variant of Golgi staining, in which pieces of central nervous tissue are immersed in a solution containing mercuric chloride or nitrate, potassium chromate and potassium dichromate. White deposits of a mercury chromate form within a small proportion of neurons and glial cells, and are converted to a black substance (probably a mixture of metallic mercury and its oxides) by subsequent immersion in an alkaline "developer" containing ammonium hydroxide.

Golgi apparatus (gol_-je‾) An organelle in eukaryotic cells consisting of stacks of flat membranous sacs that modify, store, and route products of the endoplasmic reticulum and synthesize some products, notably noncellulose carbohydrates.

gonads (go–_-nadz) The male and female sex organs; the gamete-producing organs in most animals.

growth hormone (GH) A hormone that is produced and secreted by the anterior pituitary and that has both direct (nontropic) and tropic effects on a wide variety of tissues.

gyrus - (gyri = pl.), one of the convolutions on the surface of the brain caused by infolding of the cortex.

half-life The amount of time it takes for 50% of a sample of a radioactive isotope to decay.

Harris hematoxylin. A nuclear stain based on hemalum, often used for regressive staining in routine histopathology, and progressive staining of diagnostic exfoliative cytology specimens. Hemalum comprises an acidified solution containing Al^{3+} (from aluminum ammonium sulfate) and hematein (from hematoxylin), which deposits a blue metal coordination complex on the chromatin of cell nuclei. Upon standing, the solution forms a precipitate from the ammonium alum, which must be filtered before staining. Modern Harris hematoxylin, unlike the original version, has iodate as the oxidant and acetic acid-alcohol for differentiation.

Hemalum (US) **or Haemalum** (elsewhere). A staining solution made by dissolving hematoxylin, an oxidizing agent (usually $NaIO_3$, but sometimes O_2 from the air), an aluminum salt and usually also a weak acid (acetic or citric), in water. A hydrophilic organic solvent (ethylene glycol or glycerol) is often included in the solution. The staining component is a complex of aluminum with hematein. There are many hemalum formulations; most are intended for staining cell nuclei. Synonyms: hematoxylin (in the second sense), alum-hematoxylin. See also Harris's hematoxylin, Mayer's hemalum.

Hematein (US) or **Haematein** (elsewhere). A yellow-brown compound formed by oxidation of hematoxylin, which is white when pure. Hematein forms intensely coloured dye-metal coordination complexes with aluminum, iron and other metal ions; these complexes are the colorants in staining solutions with names such as hemalum, hematoxylin, and iron hematoxylin.

Hematoxylin (US) or **Haematoxylin** (elsewhere). A phenolic compound extracted from logwood (Haematoxylum campechianum L.), a tree originally from Central America, now growing in many tropical and subtropical regions. Hematoxylin is the starting material for making many solutions that are used as biological stains. Commercial lots are available certified by the Biological Stain Commission. Preparation of most "hematoxylin" staining solutions involves oxidation to hematein, and subsequent complexation of the hematein with a metal. The hematein-metal coordination complex is the compound with specific staining properties. Both hematoxylin and hematein are included in the Colour Index name Natural black 1 (CI 75290). The name "hematoxylin" is commonly applied to solutions for which hemalum would be more appropriate; examples are Delafield's hematoxylin, Gill hematoxylin, Harris hematoxylin.

Hematoxylin and eosin (H&E). This sequence stain is the most widely used oversight stain for animal and human tissue sections, in which cell cytoplasms and nuclei are contrasted red and blue respectively. In this context hematoxylin implies hemalum, which acts as a basic dye staining nuclei and cytoplasmic ribosomes. Eosin implies eosin Y, a red acid dye which stains intra- and extracellular proteins. The abbreviation for this method has occasionally led to citation of an eponym-like name, "Hande stain".

hemoglobin (he͞-mo--glo--bin) the oxygen carrying pigment of the red blood cells (erythrocytes). It is a conjugated protein containing four heme groups and globin. A molecule of hemoglobin contains 4 globin polypeptide chains - designated alpha, beta, gamma and delta. In the adult, Hemoglobin A predominates (alpha2, beta2).

hydrogen bond A type of weak chemical bond that is formed when the slightly positive hydrogen atom of a polar covalent bond in one molecule is attracted to the slightly negative atom of a polar covalent bond in nother molecule or in another region of the same molecule.

hydrogen ion A single proton with a charge of 1_. The dissociation of a water molecule (H2O) leads to the generation of a hydroxide ion (OH–)

and a hydrogen ion (H_); in water, H_ is not found alone but associates with a watermolecule to form a hydronium ion.

Hydrogen bond. A directed, weak bond between a hydrogen atom and an adjacent electronegative atom (usually nitrogen or oxygen), there being no covalent bond between the atoms. Partial charges range from +0.15 to +0.30 on the hydrogen atoms and -0.15 to -0.50 on the electronegative atoms.

hydrolysis (hī-drol_-uh-sis) A chemical reaction that breaks bonds between two molecules by the addition of water; functions in disassembly of polymers to monomers.

hydroxide ion A water molecule that has lost a proton; OH–.

hydroxyl group (hī-drok_-sil) A chemical group consisting of an oxygen atom joined to a hydrogen atom. Molecules possessing this group are soluble in water and are called alcohols.

hyperplasia - a controlled increase in the number of normal cells in normal arrangement in an organ or tissue, causing a corresponding increase in tissue mass.

Hypertonic. Having a higher osmotic pressure than blood or extracellular fluid.

Hypotonic. Having a lower osmotic pressure than blood or extracellular fluid.

hypertrophy - an increase in individual cell size, which in turn leads to an increase in tissue mass/organ size.

hypoplasia - incomplete development or underdevelopment of a tissue, usually due to a decrease in number of cells.

hypothalamus (hī_-po–-thal_-uh-mus) The ventral part of the vertebrate forebrain; functions in maintaining homeostasis, especially in coordinating the endocrine and nervous systems; secretes hormones of the posterior pituitary and releasing factors that regulate the anterior pituitary.

insulin (in_-suh-lin) A hormone secreted by pancreatic beta cells that lowers blood glucose levels. It promotes the uptake of glucose by most body cells and the synthesis and storage of glycogen in the liver and also stimulates protein and fat synthesis.

interneuron An association neuron; a nerve cell within the central nervous system that forms synapses with sensory and/or motor neurons and integrates sensory input and motor output.

ion (ī̄_-on) An atom or group of atoms that has gained or lost one or more electrons, thus acquiring a charge.

ion channel A transmembrane protein channel that allows a specific ion to diffuse across the membrane down its concentration or electrochemical gradient.

ionic bond (ī̄_-on_-ik) A chemical bond resulting from the attraction between oppositely charged ions.

ionic compound A compound resulting from the formation of an ionic bond; also called a salt.

Iron hematoxylin. A group of stains, all of which contain or produce a metal coordination complex or complexes involving Fe^{3+} and hematein, whose precise chemical structures are uncertain. Such stains can demonstrate a variety of tissue components. Examples are Heidenhain's iron hematoxylin**,** which uses a ferric iron salt followed by naturally oxidized hematoxylin, Verhoeff's hematoxylin and Weigert's hematoxylin in which the iron oxidizes hematoxylin and bonds t.

Isosmotic. Having osmotic pressure the same as that of blood plasma or extracellular fluid.

Isotonic. Not causing shrinkage or swelling of immersed cells. An isotonic solution is typically (but not necessarily) also *isosmotic*, having the same osmotic pressure as blood plasma or extracellular fluid.

isotonic (ī̄_-so– -ton_-ik) Referring to a solution that, when surrounding a cell, causes no net movement of water into or out of the cell.

isotope (ī̄_-so– -to–p_) One of several atomic forms of an element, each with the same number of protons but a different number of neutrons, thus differing in atomic mass.

juxtamedullary nephron In mammals and birds, a nephron with a loop of Henle that extends far into the renal medulla.

kidney In vertebrates, one of a pair of excretory organs where blood filtrate is formed and processed into urine.

labia majora A pair of thick, fatty ridges that encloses and protects the rest of the vulva.

labia minora A pair of slender skin folds that surrounds the openings of the vagina and urethra.

labor A series of strong, rhythmic contractions of the uterus that expels a baby out of the uterus and vagina during childbirth.

lactation The continued production of milk from the mammary glands.

leukocyte (lū́-kō–-sīt̄) A blood cell that functions in fighting infections; also called a white blood cell.

leukocytosis - a transient increase in the number of white blood cells (leukocytes); due to various causes.

Leydig cell (lī́-dig) A cell that produces testosterone and other androgens and is located between the seminiferous tubules of the testes.

light microscope (LM) An optical instrument with lenses that refract (bend) visible light to magnify images of specimens.

lipid (lip_-id) Any of a group of large biological molecules, including fats, phospholipids, and steroids, that mix poorly, if at all, with water.

liver A large internal organ in vertebrates that performs diverse functions, such as producing bile, maintaining blood glucose level, and detoxifying poisonous chemicals in the blood.

loop of Henle The hairpin turn, with a descending and ascending limb, between the proximal and distal tubules of the vertebrate kidney; functions in water and salt reabsorption.

luteal phase That portion of the ovarian cycle during which endocrine cells of the corpus luteum secrete female hormones.

luteinizing hormone (LH) (lū́-tē̄-uh-nī́-zing) A tropic hormone that is produced and secreted by the anterior pituitary and that stimulates ovulation in females and androgen production in males.

lymph The colorless fluid, derived from interstitial fluid, in the lymphatic system of vertebrates.

lymph node An organ located along a lymph vessel. Lymph nodes filter lymph and contain cells that attack viruses and bacteria.

lymphatic system A system of vessels and nodes, separate from the circulatory system, that returns fluid, proteins, and cells to the blood.

lymphocyte A type of white blood cell that mediates immune responses. The two main classes are B cells and T cells.

lysosome (lī-suh-so–m) A membrane-enclosed sac of hydrolytic enzymes found in the cytoplasm of animal cells and some protists.

Malpighian tubule (mal-pig_-ē-un) A unique excretory organ of insects that empties into the digestive tract, removes nitrogenous wastes from the hemolymph, and functions in osmoregulation.

mammal Member of the class Mammalia, amniotes that have hair and mammary glands (glands that produce milk).

mammary gland An exocrine gland that secretes milk to nourish the young. Mammary glands are characteristic of mammals.

mast cell A vertebrate body cell that produces histamine and other molecules that trigger inflammation in response to infection and in allergic reactions.

melanocyte-stimulating hormone (MSH) A hormone produced and secreted by the anterior pituitary with multiple activities, including regulating the behavior of pigment-containing cells in the skin of some vertebrates.

melatonin A hormone that is secreted by the pineal gland and that is involved in the regulation of biological rhythms and sleep.

meninges - plural of meninx; any membrane, but specifically the three membranous coverings of the brain and spinal cord (dura mater, arachnoid and pia mater).

meningitis - inflammation of the meninges.

microscopic -- Objects or organisms that are too small to be seen with the naked eye.

microstructure -- n. In eggshell, the shape, size, orientation, and distribution of components of the shell.

midbrain One of three ancestral and embryonic regions of the vertebrate brain; develops into sensory integrating and relay centers that send sensory information to the cerebrum.

mineralocorticoid A steroid hormone secreted by the adrenal cortex that regulates salt and water homeostasis.

mitochondrion (mī̄_-to--kon_-drē̄-un) (plural, **mitochondria**) An organelle in eukaryotic cells that serves as the site of cellular respiration; uses oxygen to break down organic molecules and synthesize ATP.

molarity A common measure of solute concentration, referring to the number of moles of solute per liter of solution.

Mordant dye. (1) A dye capable of forming a metal coordination complex (e.g. hematein) or such a complex (e.g. hemalum). (2) A dye supposed by some to be bound to the tissues via dye–metal ion and metal ion–tissue bonds. (3) In the literature of histotechnology, "Mordant in..." is often an instruction to immerse slides carrying hydrated sections in a solution of a metal salt such as $FeCl_3$ or $K_2Cr_2O_7$ before staining with one or more dyes. This usage of "mordant" as a verb is sometimes incorrectly extended to other pre-staining steps, such pre-treatment with picric acid to make sections of formaldehyde-fixed tissues amenable to trichrome staining.

Mounting medium (mountant). A transparent liquid that preserves the object on a microscope slide and hardens, holding the coverslip in place. The high refractive index of the final material provides clarity to optical images of the specimen. Mountants may be resinous (organic solvent-based and permanent) or aqueous (for temporary mounts).

Mucopolysaccharide. A word seen in the literature of carbohydrate biochemistry and histochemistry before about 1970. It correctly referred to acid mucosubstances stainable with basic dyes. The word was often wrongly applied to neutral glycoproteins such as those in mucus stained with PAS.

Mucosubstances. Macromolecular carbohydrates, including polysaccharides (e.g. starch, glycogen), glycoproteins in mucus (mucins) and glycosaminoglycans in extracellular tissue components such as chondroitin sulfates in cartilage matrix and hyaluronan in softer connective tissues. Staining methods with alcian blue, the Periodic acid-Schiff reaction and labeled lectins are useful for histochemical identification of different types of mucosubstance.

Mucous. Containing, secreting or having the properties of mucus.

Mucus. Carbohydrate-rich viscous or slimy liquid that serves to protect or lubricate a surface, as in the nose, or in the alimentary tract. The physical properties of mucus are due to contained glycoproteins (stainable with

PAS) or proteoglycans (stainable with alcian blue and other basic dyes) or, commonly, to both.

necrosis - the morphological changes indicative of cell death caused by progressive enzymatic degradation.

nephron (nef̄-ron) The tubular excretory unit of the vertebrate kidney.

nerve A fiber composed primarily of the bundled axons of PNS neurons.

nerve cord -- Primary bundle of nerves in chordates, which connects the brain to the major muscles and organs of the body.

nervous system The fast-acting internal system of communication involving sensory receptors, networks of nerve cells, and connections to muscles and glands that respond to nerve signals; functions in concert with the endocrine system to effect internal regulation and maintain homeostasis.

nervous tissue Tissue made up of neurons and supportive cells.

neurohormone A molecule that is secreted by a neuron, travels in body fluids, and acts on specific target cells, changing their functioning.

neuron (nyū r̄-on) A nerve cell; the fundamental unit of the nervous system, having structure and properties that allow it to conduct signals by taking advantage of the electrical charge across its plasma membrane.

neuropeptide A relatively short chain of amino acids that serves as a neurotransmitter.

neurotransmitter A molecule that is released from the synaptic terminal of a neuron at a chemical synapse, diffuses across the synaptic cleft, and binds to the postsynaptic cell, triggering a response.

Neurosecretion. Some neurons discharge products from axonal terminals on capillary blood vessels or, in invertebrates, into the hemocoel. Examples include the peptide hormones oxytocin and vasopressin (antidiuretic hormone, ADH) which are secreted into the posterior lobe of the pituitary gland. They and their precursor/carrier proteins (neurophysins) are rich in cystine and can be demonstrated with the cysteic acid method, as can chemically similar neurosecretory materials in invertebrates.

Neutral buffered formalin (**NBF**). Generally a 10% v/v aqueous formalin solution in an approximately isotonic buffer at pH 6.8-7.4, which retards acidification by spontaneously generated formic acid, and prevents the formation of hemosiderin (formalin pigment).

Neutral dye. An old name for an ionic dye whose anion and cation are both themselves colored dyes. Romanowsky stains provide an example, in which one key component is an azure B cation and the other is an eosin Y anion. A solid neutral dye (such as Giemsa powder) is thus not non-ionic but a salt. Contrast with non-ionic dye. Synonym: neutral stain.

Neutrophil. A type of leukocyte with cytoplasmic granules that are colored purple (rather than blue or red) by Romanowsky stains.

norepinephrine A catecholamine that is chemically and functionally similar to epinephrine and acts as a hormone or neurotransmitter; also known as noradrenaline.

nuclear envelope In a eukaryotic cell, the double membrane that surrounds the nucleus, perforated with pores that regulate traffic with the cytoplasm. The outer membrane is continuous with the endoplasmic reticulum.

nuclear lamina A netlike array of protein filaments that lines the inner surface of the nuclear envelope and helps maintain the shape of the nucleus.

Nucleic acids. Linear polymers consisting of **nucleotides** joined by 3',5'-phosphodiester linkages. Deoxyribonucleic acid (DNA) encodes genes, whereas the various ribonucleic acids (RNAs) including messenger RNA (mRNA), ribosomal RNA (rRNA) and transfer RNAs (tRNAs) mediate translation and transcription of genes, resulting in synthesis of proteins.

Nucleoproteins. Basic proteins (**histones, protamines** and **ribonucleoproteins**) intimately associated with **nucleic acid** molecules.

nucleolus (nū̄-klē̄-o– -lus) (plural, **nucleoli**) A specialized structure in the nucleus, consisting of chromosomal regions containing ribosomal RNA (rRNA) genes along with ribosomal proteins imported from the cytoplasm; site of rRNA synthesis and ribosomal subunit assembly. *See also* ribosome.

nucleosome (nū̄-klē̄-o– -so–m_) The basic, beadlike unit of DNA packing in eukaryotes, consisting of a segment of DNA wound around a protein core composed of two copies of each of four types of histone.

nucleotide (nū̄_-klē̄-o–-tīd) The building block of a nucleic acid, consisting of a five-carbon sugar covalently bonded to a nitrogenous base and one or more phosphate groups.

nucleus (1) An atom's central core, containing rotons and neutrons. (2) The organelle of a eukaryotic cell that contains the genetic material in the form of chromosomes, made up of chromatin. (3) A cluster of neurons.

oocyte A cell in the female reproductive system that differentiates to form an egg.

oogenesis (o–_-uh-jen_-uh-sis) The process in the ovary that results in the production of female gametes.

oogonium (o–_-uh- go–_-nē̄-em) (plural, **oogonia**) A cell that divides mitotically to form oocytes.

organelle -- n. A membrane-bound structure in a eukaryotic cell that partitions the cell into regions which carry out different cellular functions, e.g., mitochondria, endoplasmic reticulum, lysosomes.

Osmium tetroxide. Pale yellow crystals, OsO_4, soluble in water and in non-polar solvents, but reduced to insoluble black OsO_2 by alcohol. Solid and solutions emit acrid, toxic vapor. Used mostly as a fixative (or a post-fixative following glutaraldehyde) for electron microscopy. In light microscopy OsO_4 is a stain for unsaturated lipids, which bring about reduction to black OsO_2. It is also an ingredient of traditional fixative mixtures that preserve cytoplasmic organelles such as the Golgi apparatus and mitochondria prior to embedding in paraffin and subsequent light microscopy. Synonym: Osmium(VIII) oxide.

Osmic acid is a frequently used but chemically inaccurate synonym for OsO_4, which exists as the same tetrahedral molecule in all solvents and is not an acid. Real osmate anions, $[OsO_2(OH)_4]^{2-}$, contain Os(VI) and they are formed when OsO_4 is chemically reduced at a very high pH or when Os metal is dissolved in molten KOH.

Over-dehydration. The removal of *bound water* molecules from a specimen, causing shrinkage and unwanted chemical interactions (*molecular dehydration* and *hydrophobic inversions*) among adjacent, previously insulated, molecules.

ovarian cycle (o–̄-va–r_-ē̄-un) The cyclic recurrence of the follicular phase, ovulation, and the luteal phase in the mammalian ovary, regulated by hormones.

ovary (o–_-vuh-re ̄) (1) In flowers, the portion of a carpel in which the egg-containing ovules develop. (2) In animals, the structure that produces female gametes and reproductive hormones.

oviduct (o–_-vuh-duct) A tube passing from the ovary to the vagina in invertebrates or to the uterus in vertebrates, where it is also known as a fallopian tube.

ovulation The release of an egg from an ovary. In humans, an ovarian follicle releases an egg during each uterine (menstrual) cycle.

ovule (o_-vyu ̄l) A structure that develops within the ovary of a seed plant and contains the female gametophyte.

oxytocin (ok_-si-to–_-sen) A hormone produced by the hypothalamus and released from the posterior pituitary. It induces contractions of the uterine muscles during labor and causes the mammary glands to eject milk during nursing.

pancreas (pan_-kre ̄-us) A gland with exocrine and endocrine tissues. The exocrine portion functions in digestion, secreting enzymes and an alkaline solution into the small intestine via a duct; the ductless endocrine portion functions in homeostasis, secreting the hormones insulin and glucagon into the blood.

paracrine Referring to a secreted molecule that acts on a neighboring cell.

Paraffin (wax). A mixture of long-chain (C_{20}–C_{40}) *aliphatic hydrocarbons* whose melting point is above room temperature; histological paraffin wax also contains resins or other additives to facilitate *sectioning* and *ribboning*. See also: *embedding*.

Paraformaldehyde. An insoluble, polymerized form of *formaldehyde* that can be returned to monomeric form by treatment with mild alkali. An aqueous *fixative* solution made with paraformaldehyde does not contain methanol, which is present at low concentration in a solution made by diluting *formalin*.

parathyroid hormone (PTH) A hormone secreted by the parathyroid glands that raises blood calcium level by promoting calcium release from bone and calcium retention by the kidneys.

pathology - the branch of medicine that deals with the essential nature of disease and the changes in body tissues and

Penetration. Diffusion of a liquid (*fixative* or *processing fluid*) into a tissue specimen. The rate of penetration is dependent upon whether the tissue is fresh or fixed, on the molecular size of the penetrating fluid, and on environmental factors such as agitation of the fluid, temperature, and use of vacuum. All other factors being equal, the rate of diffusion decreases as the diffusion pathway increases. A large specimen may take days or weeks before a fixative penetrates to its center.

Peroxisomes - cell structures that contain enzymes that produce hydrogen peroxide as a by-product.

Peroxidase-antiperoxidase (PAP). An antigen-antibody complex in which three molecules of HRP are bound to the Fab segments of two molecules of immunoglobulin that are antibodies to HRP. The two Fc segments of PAP are free to combine with Fab segments of an unlabeled secondary antibody to immunoglobulin of the species in which both the primary antibody and the anti-HRP were raised. Sites of bound PAP are made visible with a histochemical reaction for peroxidase activity.

peptide - a protein with a small number of amino acids.

perfusion - transport of blood through blood vessels from heart to internal organs, tissues, etc.

pH. The logarithm (to base 10) of the reciprocal of the concentration (in molar terms) of hydrogen ions (protons) in water that contains dissolved substances: $pH = -\log[H^+]$. Solutions with low pH are acidic; those with high pH are alkaline. The pH of perfectly pure water is 7.0. Ordinary distilled or otherwise purified water has pH 5-6, owing to acidification by carbon dioxide taken up from the atmosphere. Because of the logarithmic nature of the scale, a solution at pH 2 is ten times more acidic than one at pH 3, and a hundred times more acidic than one at pH 4.

pH A measure of hydrogen ion concentration equal to $-\log [H\_]$ and ranging in value from 0 to 14.

Picric acid. A small acid dye of the nitro class. Used in polychrome stains as the cytoplasmic staining component in mixtures with acid fuchsine (Van Gieson's stain) or with other dyes, including aniline blue and sirius red F3B. Has also been used as a coagulative fixative, notably in Bouin's fluid. Picric acid is conveniently kept as a saturated aqueous solution (1.28% w/v); it is more soluble in ethanol (8.3%) and other organic solvents. Synonyms: CI 10305, trinitrophenol. Hazard warning: solid picric acid must be stored under water because it explodes if its temperature reaches

300°C, which could arise from friction of dry powder in the thread of a screw-cap jar.

pineal gland (pī̄-nē̄-ul) A small gland on the dorsal surface of the vertebrate forebrain that secretes the hormone melatonin.

pituitary gland (puh-tū̄-uh-ta–r_-ē̄) An endocrine gland at the base of the hypothalamus; consists of a posterior lobe, which stores and releases two hormones produced by the hypothalamus, and an anterior lobe, which produces and secretes many hormones that regulate diverse body functions.

pleura (pleural = adj.) - the serous membrane covering the lungs and lining the walls of the thoracic cavity; the two layers thus enclose a potential space - the pleural cavity.

posterior pituitary An extension of the hypothalamus composed of nervous tissue that secretes oxytocin and antidiuretic hormone made in the hypothalamus; a temporary storage site for these hormones.

Preservation. Protection of specimens from destruction by either making the environment hypertonic with sugar or salts, by changing their molecular structure (fixation), or by freezing.

primary oocyte (o–_-uh-sī̄t) An oocyte prior to completion of meiosis I.

Probe. A fluorescent compound used for vital staining. Synonym: fluorescent probe.

Processing fluid. Any of various solvents used to prepare fixed, aqueous tissue specimens for infiltration with non-aqueous embedding media. Most typically, processing fluids include a graded series of ethanol (70%, 80%, 95% and 100%) as dehydrants followed by a clearing agent.

Progressive staining. Selective coloration of a specimen resulting from the staining of an initially colorless tissue preparation until the required staining intensity and staining pattern is achieved. Romanowsky stains are usually used progressively, with staining continued until purple nuclei are obtained. Contrast with regressive staining.

progesterone A steroid hormone that prepares the uterus for pregnancy; the major progestin in mammals.

Prokaryotes - single-celled organisms that are the earliest and most primitive forms of life on earth.

progestin Any steroid hormone with progesteronelike activity.

prolactin A hormone produced and secreted by the anterior pituitary with a great diversity of effects in different vertebrate species. In mammals, it stimulates growth of and milk production by the mammary glands.

prostate gland (pros_-ta–t) A gland in human males that secretes an acid-neutralizing component of semen.

pyknosis - a thickening, especially degeneration of a cell in which the nucleus shrinks in size and the chromatin condenses to a solid, structureless mass.

Quinone. An oxidation product of an *ortho-* or *para-*diphenol. As commonly formulated, oxygen atoms are doubly bonded to adjacent or opposite carbon atoms of a 6-membered ring that also has double bonds between the pairs of carbon atoms not joined to oxygen. Although double and single bonds alternate throughout the molecule (making a *conjugated system*), a quinone's ring is not aromatic, like that of a phenol or an aromatic hydrocarbon.

Quinonoid. The appearance of rings of *conjugated* carbon atoms, similar to those of *quinones*, in the usual structural formulae of many *dyes* and other colored organic compounds. Quinonoid compounds absorb light of longer (visible) wavelength than compounds with aromatic ring systems of comparable size and structure.

renal cortex The outer portion of the vertebrate kidney.

renal medulla The inner portion of the vertebrate kidney, beneath the renal cortex.

Regressive staining. Selective coloration of a specimen resulting from *differentiating* an initially over-stained tissue preparation until the required staining intensity and staining pattern are achieved. *Harris's hematoxylin* is used regressively in many histopathology laboratories. Contrast with *progressive staining*.

renal pelvis The funnel-shaped chamber that receives processed filtrate from the vertebrate kidney's collecting ducts and is drained by the ureter.

renin-angiotensin-aldosterone system (RAAS) A hormone cascade pathway that helps regulate blood pressure and blood volume.

Resolution. The shortest distance apart for two different points to be seen as visibly separate. With an ideal light microscope using an apochromatic oil immersion objective of high numerical aperture, diffraction limits this separation to about 200 nm (0.2 μm). In routine work there is blurring of detail in areas less than 1 μm across, but strongly stained smaller objects, such as bacteria, may nevertheless be seen. Ultraviolet microscopy (seldom used) and *confocal microscopy* provide resolution to 100 nm, and several types of super-resolution microscopy allow resolution to 20 nm. The *electron microscope* provides, with biological specimens, resolution to the level of *macromolecules* (1 nm) but it is poorly suited to the collection of histochemical data. The atomic force microscope can image individual atoms (0.1–0.5 nm) on some surfaces.

ribosome (rī̄_-buh-so–m_) A complex of rRNA and protein molecules that functions as a site of protein synthesis in the cytoplasm; consists of a large and a small subunit. In eukaryotic cells, each subunit is assembled in the nucleolus.

rough ER That portion of the endoplasmic reticulum with ribosomes attached.

Saline. Immunological reagents are usually dissolved in a solution of sodium chloride, 0.7–0.9% in a buffer (such as 0.03 M phosphate) at pH 7.2–7.4. Phosphate-buffered saline is commonly called PBS. As a solvent in immunostaining procedures, saline may optionally also contain a surfactant to enhance penetration of immunoglobulin reagents, and also an indifferent protein (such as albumin or casein) to compete with the antibody for nonspecific (weak) binding to substances other than the intended antigen. PBS is not always the ideal diluent, especially for monoclonal antibodies, which often give superior results when applied at a pH above and below the usual range, without added NaCl.

Salt. A compound in which a metal or other cation is neutralized by an anion.

scrotum A pouch of skin outside the abdomen that houses the testes; functions in maintaining the testes at the lower temperature required for spermatogenesis.

secondary oocyte (o–_-uh-sī̄ t) An oocyte that has completed the first of the two meiotic divisions.

sensory neuron A nerve cell that receives information from the internal or external environment and transmits signals to the central nervous system.

sensory receptor An organ, cell, or structure within a cell that responds to specific stimuli from an organism's external or internal environment.

serotonin (ser_-uh-to–_-nin) A neurotransmitter, synthesized from the amino acid tryptophan, that functions in the central nervous system.

Serum. Blood *plasma* from which the fibrinogen has been removed. Whole blood is centrifuged, after clotting and shrinkage of the clot. Mammalian sera contain about 8% w/v protein, consisting of approximately equal proportions of *albumin* and *globulin*.

Shrinkage (of specimens). Occurs in insufficiently fixed specimens when aggressive dehydrants (e.g., ethanol), remove bound water from macromolecules, allowing intra- and inter-molecular interactions (ionic and hydrogen bonding, as well as van der Waals forces) between once-insulated chemical groups.

smooth ER That portion of the endoplasmic reticulum that is free of ribosomes.

sodium-potassium pump A transport protein in the plasma membrane of animal cells that actively transports sodium out of the cell and potassium into the cell.

Specificity of staining. The staining of a single cell or tissue component, and no other. Specific stains are much less common than many believe. Even a reagent such as a labeled antibody often gives positive artifacts, due to non-immunological staining mechanisms. Contrary to common parlance, there is no such thing as "quite specific"; that phrase and its equivalents actually refer to selective staining. See also selectivity of staining and sensitivity of staining.

Staining. Visual labeling of some cell or tissue entity (anything from a molecular fragment to a physiological process) by attaching or depositing in its vicinity a visual marker of characteristic color or shape. The term most commonly (but not exclusively) refers to the use of a solution of a dye to color a biological specimen. The transfer of dye from solution to specimen does not usually require any change in covalent bonds or oxidation state, although there are exceptions (e.g., Schiff reagent). Other types of staining include localization of pigments and mineral deposits in tissues, enzyme histochemistry and immunohistochemistry.

spermatogenesis The continuous and prolific production of mature sperm cells in the testis.

spermatogonium (plural, **spermatogonia**) A cell that divides mitotically to form spermatocytes.

squamous (cells) - cell type often seen in areas exposed to significant irritation or trauma - e.g. skin.

steroid A type of lipid characterized by a carbon skeleton consisting of four fused rings with various chemical groups attached.

subcutaneous (s.c. or SQ) - beneath the skin.

synapse (sin_-aps) The junction where a neuron communicates with another cell across a narrow gap via a neurotransmitter or an electrical coupling.

testis (plural, **testes**) The male reproductive organ, or gonad, in which sperm and reproductive hormones are produced.

testosterone A steroid hormone required for development of the male reproductive system, spermatogenesis, and male secondary sex characteristics; the major androgen in mammals.

thymus (thī_-mus) A small organ in the thoracic cavity of vertebrates where maturation of T cells is completed.

thyroid gland An endocrine gland, located on the ventral surface of the trachea, that secretes two iodine-containing hormones, triiodothyronine (T3) and thyroxine (T4), as well as calcitonin.

thyroxine (T4) One of two iodine-containing hormones that are secreted by the thyroid gland and that help regulate metabolism, development, and maturation in vertebrates.

tissue An integrated group of cells with a common structure, function, or both.

Tissue processing. The sequence of steps starting from a fresh specimen and culminating in the formation of an embedded tissue block. Major stages usually include fixation, dehydration, clearing and infiltration with paraffin wax or other embedding media. Tissue processing may be accomplished by hand, but in larger laboratories it is achieved using a mechanical device (tissue processor). See also Processing fluids.

Tissue processor. A mechanical device that sequentially exposes specimens to the various fluids involved with tissue processing. The device may allow application of pressure, vacuum, heat or agitation to the fluids to hasten processing time.

Tissue section. A thin slice cut off the face of a specimen, usually by use of a microtome. A paraffin section comes from a specimen embedded in paraffin wax, a plastic section comes from one embedded in a plastic embedding medium, and a frozen section has been cut from a frozen tissue block, usually with a cryostat. Before staining, paraffin sections are dewaxed and methylmethacrylate plastic sections have their resin removed. Glycol methacrylate and epoxy plastic sections are routinely stained with the resin remaining in situ. Contrast with smear.

transformation (1) The conversion of a normal animal cell to a cancerous cell. (2) A change in genotype and phenotype due to the assimilation of external DNA by a cell. When the external DNA is from a member of a different species, transformation results in horizontal gene transfer.

transmission The passage of a nerve impulse along axons.

transmission electron microscope (TEM) A microscope that passes an electron beam through very thin sections stained with metal atoms and is primarily used to study the internal ultrastructure of cells.

transport vesicle A small membranous sac in a eukaryotic cell's cytoplasm carrying molecules produced by the cell.

triiodothyronine (T3) (trī̄_-ī̄ -o–_-do– -thī̄_-ro– -nē̄ n) One of two iodine-containing hormones that are secreted by the thyroid gland and that help regulate metabolism, development, and maturation in vertebrates.

tropic hormone A hormone that has an endocrine gland or cells as a target.

ultrastructure -- The detailed structure of a specimen, such as a cell, tissue, or organ, that can be observed only by electron microscopy. Also called fine structure. In eggshell, ultrastructure refers to the three-dimensional arrangement of mineral crystals and organic matter. It is described in terms of calcite or aragonite mineralogy and the transition between different zones of organization within the shell. Distinct zones of organization are called ultrastructure zones.

uterus A female organ where eggs are fertilized and/or development of the young occurs.

vagina Part of the female reproductive system between the uterus and the outside opening; the birth canal in mammals. During copulation, the vagina accommodates the male's penis and receives sperm.

vas deferens In mammals, the tube in the male reproductive system in which sperm travel from the epididymis to the urethra.

vasa recta The capillary system in the kidney that serves the loop of Henle.

vesicle (ves_-i-kul) A membranous sac in the cytoplasm of a eukaryotic cell.

Dr. Chanchal Kumar Manna, was a Professor of Zoology, University of Kalyani, Kalyani 741235, Nadia, W.B., INDIA. At present he has retired from services. During the long Scientific career and for the benefit of the students, Professor Manna was interested in studying various aspects of Histophysiology, Immunocytochemistry, Molecular Biology, Behavioral Biology, Ultra structural and Ethno medicinal Research. For these specific reasons he has to travel in various reputed Scientific Laboratories e.g., Institute of Molecular Biology, Taipei, Taiwan R.O.C.; Nara Women's University, Nara, Japan ; Institute of Molecular Biology, Salya Campus, Mahidol University, Bangkok , Thailand , and Bhaba Atomic Research Centre, Mumbai .

In addition to his Teaching assignments, Dr. Manna was interested in conducting Research.

Within limited resources he has guided many students for the award of the Ph.D. degree. For this purpose and he has to set up a Laboratory to do some work on Histophysiology, Comparative Anatomy, Molecular Biology, Behavioral Biology and Ethno medicinal Research. Many Research students have got their Ph.D. degree and working in their separate fields.

At present Professor Manna is interested to write some Books which will be used by the Research Students and other workers in the field of Biology, Medical Physiology and Ethnomedicine Research.

www.ingramcontent.com/pod-product-compliance
Lightning Source LLC
Chambersburg PA
CBHW040516220526
45473CB00012B/2875